SINGLE-CASE RESEARCH METHODS IN SPORT AND EXERCISE PSYCHOLOGY

Single-case research is a powerful method for examining change in outcome variables such as behaviour, performance and psychological constructs, and for assessing the efficacy of interventions. It has innumerable uses within the context of sport and exercise science/psychology, such as in the development of more effective performance techniques for athletes and sportspeople and in helping us to better understand exercise behaviours in clinical populations. However, the fundamental principles and techniques of single-case research have not always been clearly understood by students and researchers working in these fields.

Single-Case Research Methods in Sport and Exercise Psychology is the first book to fully explain single-case research in the context of sport and exercise. Starting with first principles, the book offers a comprehensive introduction to the single-case research process, from study design to data analysis and presentation. Including examples from across sport and exercise psychology, the book provides practical guidance for students and researchers and demonstrates the advantages and common pitfalls of single-case research for anybody working in applied or behavioural science in a sport or exercise setting.

Jamie Barker is Senior Lecturer in Sport and Exercise Psychology in the Department of Sport and Exercise, Staffordshire University, UK.

Paul McCarthy is a Lecturer in Psychology in the Department of Psychology, Glasgow Caledonian University, UK.

Marc Jones is Reader in Sport and Exercise Psychology in the Department of Sport and Exercise, Staffordshire University, UK.

Aidan Moran is Professor of Cognitive Psychology and Director of the Psychology Research Laboratory at University College Dublin, Republic of Ireland.

SINGLE-CASE RESEARCH METHODS IN SPORT AND EXERCISE PSYCHOLOGY

*Jamie Barker, Paul McCarthy,
Marc Jones and Aidan Moran*

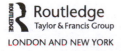

Routledge
Taylor & Francis Group

LONDON AND NEW YORK

First published 2011
by Routledge
2 Park Square, Milton Park, Abingdon, Oxon, OX14 4RN

Simultaneously published in the USA and Canada
by Routledge
711 Third Avenue, New York, NY 10017

Routledge is an imprint of the Taylor & Francis Group, an informa business

LEEDS TRINITY UNIVERSITY

British Library Cataloguing in Publication Data
A catalogue record for this book is available from the British Library

Library of Congress Cataloging in Publication Data
Single case research methods in sport and exercise psychology/by Jamie
Barker. . . [et al.].
p. cm.
1. Sports–Psychological aspects. 2. Sports psychology. 3. Sports injuries–
Psychological aspects. 4. Exercise–Psychological aspects. 5. Sports
medicine. I. Barker, Jamie.
GV706.4.S544 2011
796.01–dc22
2010041818

ISBN: 978-0-415-56511-0 (hbk)
ISBN: 978-0-415-56512-7 (pbk)
ISBN: 978-0-203-86188-2 (ebk)

Typeset in Bembo by Prepress Projects Ltd, Perth, UK

For Emma, Lucy, Mum and Dad, with love – Jamie

For Lesley and Liam, for all time – Paul

To Helen, Molly and the rest of my family, for all your love and support – Marc

To Angela and Kevin, with all my love – Aidan

CONTENTS

ILLUSTRATIONS

Figures

Tables

FOREWORD

As an academic and practitioner interested in promoting applied research, the arrival of a resource dedicated to the execution of rigorous, professional single-case research could not be timelier. In the British academic sector we are entering an era in which the 'impact' of our research is becoming more closely evaluated, and academics will simply be held more accountable to the 'So what?' question. One of the criticisms that could be levelled at current research within sport psychology is that too few studies focus on interventions – a scenario that automatically decelerates the progress of the field and deteriorates relationships with coaches and practitioners who want to know what works, why and how. Questions such as 'What behaviour change will this intervention make?' or 'Do these psychological techniques and/or processes yield changes that are retained over time?' are fairly fundamental to the stakeholders on the ground. Therefore, it is important for academic researchers to take on more responsibility for helping with the answers.

At a personal level, I became intrigued by the possibilities afforded by single-case research in the context of determining if the relatively stable, 'less than positive' achievement goal profiles of a small group of talented young tennis players could be influenced by an individualized player–coach–parent intervention programme (Harwood and Swain 2002). To be meaningful and ecologically rich, the intervention took place in natural training and tournament contexts, and it was labour intensive in supporting each individual player, coach and parent with educational tasks and reinforcement over a prolonged period. The nature of the sample and intervention did not lend itself to a group-based design, but a multiple-baseline across-participants design offered a valuable alternative that ultimately helped achievement goal researchers and coaches to be confident that social cognitions could be positively influenced by a co-ordinated environmental approach.

As always, there were limitations in the aforementioned study and I suspect that some of these may have been alleviated if there had been a detailed textbook focused entirely on the nuts and bolts of single-case research in sport and exercise settings. Confidence and perception are major factors in this respect. It is important to be confident that you have covered all of the features of sound single-case research and truly understand what you are doing and why you are doing it (e.g., establishing the most suitable design for your study – A–B; A–B plus retention; A–B–A–B; baseline assessment and stability; implementing the stagger; the logistics of multiple treatments; visual inspection and trend analysis; the process of social validation). Gaining this increased confidence enables you to overcome the often-misguided perception that single-case research is not scientific. Indeed, it attempts to optimize control but in the context of endeavouring not to overly interrupt the existing 'real-world goings on'. This book offers the reader an opportunity to become more confident, knowledgeable and reassured about single-case designs, and most importantly I think that it will encourage the reader to conduct more practically valuable work that will raise the profile of the discipline.

As a specialist research methods text, the authors have organized the book in a very logical and systematic manner. The opening chapters champion the relevance and applicability of single-case research (with published examples) and offer a historical appreciation of the differing research methods that have led to the development of single-case designs. The general features, validity issues and cardinal principles of single-case research are then introduced before going into greater detail about each phase of the research process itself. The 'engine room' of the book focuses on the variety of design variations that it is possible to implement, from the more traditional multiple-baseline designs to the more intricate 'changing-criterion' and 'alternating-treatments' designs. In each chapter the varying designs are explained with evidence-based illustrations from mainstream and sport research, and are evaluated with their strengths and limitations to inform the reader. Hypothetical and real applied cases from sport and exercise nicely contextualize each chapter and orient the reader to what topic is to follow. This is nicely illustrated within the chapter on data analysis in which attention is given to how changes in the targeted variables (including behaviour) are evaluated. The more traditional use of visual inspection techniques is appraised alongside the possibilities for statistical evaluation and trend analysis of the data. Care is afforded to reinforce the difference between statistical significance and the clinical or applied significance of changes brought about by an intervention. As a practitioner working with elite-level athletes, this aspect is particularly salient given that small numerical improvements can mean much larger effects on a number of different levels.

Whether you are an undergraduate or postgraduate attempting your first piece of intervention research, a seasoned academic trying to apply your research area to the real world or a consultant focused on determining the effectiveness of your work, you'll find a wealth of ideas and processes in this book that will strengthen your respective projects. Enjoy the journey!

Chris Harwood, PhD, C. Psychol
Reader in Applied Sport Psychology
Loughborough University, UK

PREFACE

The seminal work of Kazdin (1982) and Barlow and Hersen (1984) into single-case research methods has prompted repeated calls for sport and exercise researchers and practitioners to adopt these methods into their practice (e.g., Bryan 1987; Hrycaiko and Martin 1996; Smith 1988). These calls seem appropriate on a number of levels. First, demonstrating consultancy effectiveness or accountability is a key component of many accreditation programmes (e.g., British Psychological Society; British Association of Sport and Exercise Sciences), professional practice and applied research. Second, other applied domains (e.g., psychology, occupational and physical therapy, social work) embraced single-case research methods many years ago. Despite the obvious justification for single-case research becoming more prominent in sport and exercise psychology, many undergraduate, postgraduate and accreditation programmes do not provide sufficient education to students about these methods. One reason for this lack of education could be because a specific text documenting how to integrate single-case methods into sport and exercise settings has not been available. The lack of a specific text has prompted much frustration and discussion amongst the four of us as applied behavioural practitioners and researchers. Regularly over recent times have we found ourselves searching for sport and exercise examples to pass onto students, when reaching for a text that included such detail would have helped them to understand the methods more thoroughly. Therefore, long overdue in our eyes, we present *Single-Case Research Methods in Sport and Exercise Psychology*. We intend this text to be a useful resource for students, scientists and practitioners in increasing their awareness and providing a guide through the main facets of using single-case research methods in their applied practice and research. Therefore, the primary purpose of this text is to provide a resource of single-case designs, procedures and analysis strategies. We hope you enjoy our story!

Jamie Barker
Paul McCarthy
Marc Jones
Aidan Moran

ACKNOWLEDGEMENTS

To our families and friends we express our deep appreciation for their unquestionable love and support during the compilation of this book. To Dr Chris Harwood we extend our sincere gratitude for his kind and supportive words in the foreword. We are fortunate to have worked with many supportive and professional individuals at Routledge and we are particularly thankful to Joshua Wells and Simon Whitmore in helping us to get the idea off the ground and seeing us through to the end. Finally, we express our thanks to Springer, Sage, the American Psychological Association, Wiley and Sons, Elsevier, the *Journal of Applied Behaviour Analysis*, Taylor and Francis and Human Kinetics for their co-operation and assistance in granting permission to use copyright material.

1

INTRODUCTION TO SINGLE-CASE RESEARCH

An overview

In this chapter, we will:

- introduce the concept of single-case research designs in sport and exercise;
- describe different single-case research designs in sport and exercise;
- describe how single-case research designs can contribute to research and practice in sport and exercise.

Introduction

The purpose of research is to increase knowledge (Clark-Carter 2009). This book presents one type of research design for sport and exercise scientists and practitioners to fulfil that objective: single-case research designs. Single-case research designs can complement and extend a sport and exercise literature that relies generally on traditional group designs. In this book, single-case research designs are discussed primarily from a psychological perspective, which is in keeping with most literature on single-case research designs and our background as sport and exercise psychologists. However, the principles and guidelines outlined can be applied to other domains in sport and exercise, such as coaching, biomechanics, physiology and nutrition.

To begin this book, this chapter explains what we mean by 'single-case research designs', introduces the different types of designs and provides examples of these designs in understanding human behaviour generally and sport and exercise specifically. We finish by outlining when single-case research designs can be useful in sport and exercise contexts.

What is single-case research?

In single-case research, data are typically collected from one participant. The researcher is interested in exploring what changes occur in response to the manipulation of one or more variables. For example, a tennis coach may be interested in the influence of positive feedback on her player's confidence levels, or a psychologist may be interested in the influence of a psychological skills package comprising imagery and positive self-talk on the anxiety levels of a junior sprinter. There are variations of this typical model. For example, rather than collecting data from a single participant, the focus may be on investigating outcomes at a group level. The single case in this example would be an identifiable group such as a sports team or exercise class. To illustrate, an exercise leader may choose to explore whether or not offering incentives to attend an exercise class increases attendance. Sometimes a multiple-baseline design is used (see Chapter 6) in which data from more than one participant (usually about three or four) are reported separately. If the participants demonstrate similar changes in response to the variable or variables manipulated (i.e., each case looks similar) it strengthens the conclusions that the researchers can draw from the data because of the replication of effects. Although there are variations in the type of design that can be employed, a single-case research design is usually about what happens to *one* person. It is this reliance on data from single individuals that makes single-case research problematic for some scientists and practitioners – especially those trained in the logic of group comparisons. Yet in this book, we aim to demonstrate that single-case research designs can make a significant contribution to sport and exercise literature. More precisely, over the coming chapters we intend to explain *why*, and show *how*, single-case research designs can be effectively, rigorously and scientifically used in sport and exercise settings. In doing so, we seek to extend the original contributions to this area in the 1980s and 1990s, made most noticeably by Bryan (1987), Hrycaiko and Martin (1996), Jones (1996), Mace (1990) and Smith (1988).

Before we describe what single-case research actually is, we will briefly discuss case studies. Case studies are often mistaken for single-case research; however, in a case study observations are made under uncontrolled and unsystematic conditions (Brossart, Meythaler, Parker, McNamara and Elliot 2008; Goode and Hatt 1952). Away from the academic literature, many people in sport and exercise settings intuitively use a case-study approach. For example, in an effort to increase his knowledge of elite teams' training methods, the football manager, Roy Keane, went to New Zealand in the summer of 2008 to observe how the All Blacks rugby team prepared for competitive games. Case studies also abound in exercise settings with numerous examples in the popular media and in the advertising literature of gymnasia providing case studies of individuals who have benefited from increasing their exercise activity. This shows that many people believe that case studies can enlighten and motivate. In short, the informal study of individuals and organizations as case studies may be used to illustrate understanding and development in sport and exercise.

Case studies of individuals are also well represented in the scientific literature. Indeed, they have stimulated current understanding of human behaviour and functioning. For example, many psychology students are aware of the consequences of a horrific accident suffered by a man named Phineas Gage in 1848 (see Macmillan 2000). He was working as a construction foreman when an accidental explosion propelled an iron rod under his left cheekbone, through his frontal cortex and out through the top of his skull. The subsequent change in Phineas Gage's personality, particularly his impaired social skills, illustrated the important role that the frontal cortex played in social activity. The case study describes an event and outcome but does not enable the experimenter to control any of the variables involved. An interesting example of a case study in sport and exercise comes from the work of Vealey and Walter (1994), who interviewed the Olympic archer, Darrell Pace, about his approach to competition. This case study about a successful Olympic athlete yielded some valuable information on important aspects such as the type of training regimes that are most effective, what psychological strategies might help performance in competition and how these psychological aspects might be developed. Although interesting, it is a descriptive case study and it is impossible to determine with certainty which aspects were instrumental in helping Darrell Pace achieve Olympic success.

Case studies can also describe an intervention carried out to produce a desired change. An example of a case study in sport is the work of Mace, Eastman and Carroll (1987) with an Olympic gymnast. Figure 1.1 reveals the main essence of the study.

The case study reported by Mace et al. (1987) is appealing because it outlines how to apply a psychological intervention to help a high-level athlete. Of particular interest is the way in which the intervention is structured, comprising an education phase (session 1), a skill acquisition phase (sessions 2–6) and an application phase (sessions 7–12). This illustrates how psychological skills can be introduced, acquired and transferred to the competitive arena. In that sense it is a useful paper because it illustrates how psychological skills training can be delivered in an applied setting. However, as with all studies, it has certain limitations. For example, it is not possible to determine unequivocally from the case study if it was the *intervention* that resulted in the positive change and, if so, what the nature of that change was. Also, no measures of anxiety were taken. There was no formal comparison of competition performance scores from before and after the intervention to resolve whether the techniques employed actually produced a meaningful change. In short, Mace et al.'s (1987) study lacks objective pre- and post-intervention data and that makes it difficult to accurately determine the effect of the intervention.

To summarize, case studies are often mistaken for single-case research but they lack the control and rigour that enable definite conclusions to be drawn from the data. It is not that case studies cannot illustrate, educate, enlighten,

A male Olympic gymnast was very anxious about performing on the pommelled horse in competition and frequently fell off. Mace et al. (1987) reported the use of a stress inoculation training programme comprising relaxation, imagery and positive self-talk to help the gymnast overcome his difficulties. The sessions were as follows:

- Session 1: An education session about the effects of anxiety on performance.
- Session 2: The gymnast was taught a relaxation technique and visualized himself performing the voluntary routines on all the Olympic apparatus except the pommelled horse.
- Session 3: The content of session 2 was repeated and training in the use of self-talk provided.
- Session 4: The session involved relaxation training and visualizing another international gymnast performing his routine perfectly.
- Sessions 5 and 6: The gymnast visualized himself performing the pommelled horse routine successfully and engaging in positive self-talk.
- Sessions 7–10: The gymnast was asked to use the skills before performing the pommelled horse routine in the gymnasium.
- Session 11: The gymnast performed the pommelled horse routine in front of his fellow national squad members.
- Session 12: The gymnast performed the routine in an informal competition organized by his coach.

Following the intervention the gymnast performed well in two subsequent competitions and reported that the intervention had been successful in helping him overcome his difficulties.

FIGURE 1.1 Stress inoculation and gymnastics.

interest or motivate. They can. But because they lack control and rigour, the conclusions that they generate are limited, and by themselves they cannot be considered to satisfy the highest standards of scientific research. However, as we shall now explain, it *is* possible to conduct research with a single participant and that is the focus of the remainder of the book.

Single-case research designs

As we have just explained, case studies are descriptive methods and lack sufficient experimental control to exclude the threats to internal and external validity (see explanations of these terms in Chapter 9). In that sense, a case study cannot be considered a research design; however, it is possible to bring rigour to research with one participant. For example, Ebbinghaus, a German psychologist, provided some of the earliest studies of memory (Ebbinghaus 1964). He explored the factors influencing the recall of nonsense syllables (e.g., 'juz', 'gof'). Although Ebbinghaus manipulated the variables of interest (e.g., amount of nonsense syllables), and rigorously recorded the outcome (e.g., time taken to learn the syllables), the data were collected from one participant – himself. Clearly, Ebbinghaus' seminal research yielded fundamental principles of memory that are still, in general, accepted today (Morgan and Morgan 2001). In research with a single participant (or group) it is possible to have similar rigour to that used in experimental designs in which a control group is compared on performance with experimental group(s). These more rigorous studies are called single-case research and it is these designs that are the focus of this book. Using a single-case research design, a researcher can control the independent variable(s) or introduce an intervention and examine the influence on the dependent variable(s). Throughout the book we often refer to dependent variables as target variables. In this section we describe the different types of design in single-case research.

To illustrate how a single-case research design can be applied in sport and exercise, an athlete's target variable (e.g., behaviour, or psychological response) is measured repeatedly, and a baseline established, so that trends and changes in the data can be examined as the treatment is introduced, and even possibly withdrawn (Kratochwill, Mott and Dodson 1984). In effect, the participant acts as his or her own control by comparing changes following the intervention to the baseline (control) phase. One common design is an A–B design in which the variable of interest (e.g., performance, or a psychological construct such as anxiety) is recorded during a baseline phase (A) and compared with that recorded after the intervention (B). For example, a psychologist interested in applying a relaxation technique to help a young athlete cope with the pressure of competition may record her anxiety over a series of eight competitions before administering the intervention and monitoring anxiety levels in a subsequent eight competitions. An example of an A–B design is shown in Figures 1.2–1.6 in which Barker and Jones (2008) reported the effects of a hypnosis intervention to enhance mood and self-efficacy in a professional soccer player.

One potential problem with an A–B design is that it is possible that any observed differences may be a consequence of maturation (i.e., normal development) and, hence, may not be caused by the intervention used. Designs in which the intervention is withdrawn (A–B–A; see Chapter 5) or withdrawn and then re-introduced (A–B–A–B; see Chapter 5) can also be used. If the variable of interest changes in line with the introduction or withdrawal of the intervention then it is possible to have confidence that the changes occurred because of the intervention. For example, a rugby coach may be interested in exploring if providing individualized feedback on a player's performance after each game increases game involvement. The coach hypothesizes that individual feedback will reduce the tendency for this player to 'coast' during games and increase

A professional soccer player reported low self-efficacy and a negative mood state relative to his soccer performance. To assess the participant data were collected from interviews; a measure of trait sport confidence, a measure of self-efficacy and a measure of mood were completed fifteen minutes before each game; and a self-reported measure of performance was made after the game. The data from the self-efficacy, mood and performance measures were collected from eight games before the intervention was delivered. This meant that Barker and Jones (2008) had a good idea of how the participant typically felt before competition and how he performed during competition and, crucially, it provided data against which it would be possible to compare any changes after the intervention had taken place. The intervention pro-gramme consisted of eight hypnosis sessions. These sessions comprised the presentation of ego-strengthening suggestions. As soon as the intervention started, data on self-efficacy, mood and performance were collected from a further eight games and a measure of trait confidence and further interviews conducted. Both visual and statistical analysis (see Chapter 9 for more detail on this approach) revealed substantial increases in trait sport confidence, self-efficacy, positive affect and soccer performance, as well as a substantial decrease in negative affect over the course of the intervention. The findings of this case study suggested that hypnosis can be used to enhance self-efficacy, affect and sport performance (Figures 1.3–1.6).

FIGURE 1.2 Hypnosis and soccer performance.

the tendency to maintain effort. Game involvement may be assessed by a pre-determined set of criteria (e.g., number of passes, tackles, line breaks). Baseline performance could be monitored for a number of games, the individual feedback introduced for a period, then removed and then re-introduced. If game involve-ment increases when the individual feedback is introduced, reduces when it is removed and increases when it is re-introduced then individual feedback would appear to be associated with increased game involvement.

With some interventions (e.g., those in which the participant is asked to use a particular psychological technique or learn a particular behaviour), this may not always be possible. To illustrate, it may be difficult following a cognitive restructuring intervention (i.e., the participant is trained systematically to think about some aspect of his or her game in a more constructive manner), such as in a case in which a field hockey player addresses her aggressive behaviour towards umpires. After the intervention, the player may recognize that, because umpires do not change decisions, complaining is futile. So it would be difficult in this circumstance to ask the hockey player to return her thought processes to the way they were before the intervention and behave accordingly. Also, if an

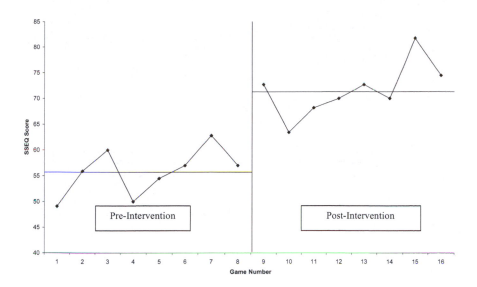

FIGURE 1.3 Pre- and post-intervention soccer self-efficacy. Reprinted with permission from J. B. Barker and M. V. Jones (2008) The effects of hypnosis on self-efficacy, affect, and soccer performance: A case study. *Journal of Clinical Sport Psychology, 2*, 127–147.

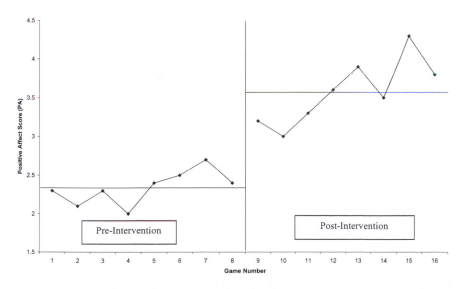

FIGURE 1.4 Pre- and post-intervention positive affect scores. Reprinted with permission from J. B. Barker and M. V. Jones (2008) The effects of hypnosis on self-efficacy, affect, and soccer performance: A case study. *Journal of Clinical Sport Psychology, 2*, 127–147.

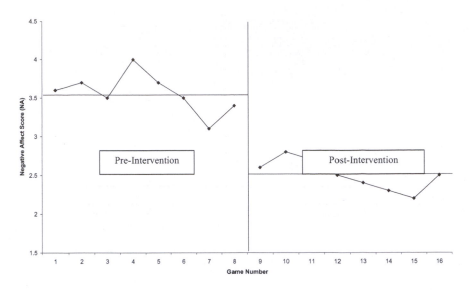

FIGURE 1.5 Psychometric data collected from a professional soccer player. Reprinted with permission from J. B. Barker and M. V. Jones (2008) The effects of hypnosis on self-efficacy, affect, and soccer performance: A case study. *Journal of Clinical Sport Psychology, 2,* 127–147.

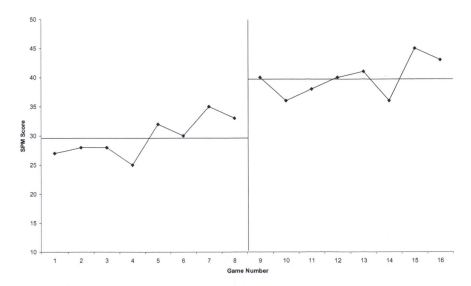

FIGURE 1.6 Pre- and post-intervention soccer performance scores. Reprinted with permission from J. B. Barker and M. V. Jones (2008) The effects of hypnosis on self-efficacy, affect, and soccer performance: A case study. *Journal of Clinical Sport Psychology, 2,* 127–147.

intervention is successful, an athlete may not want to stop using a strategy that is helping him or her perform well. For example, an athlete may not want to stop using a relaxation strategy that he or she perceives is useful. Nevertheless, there are illustrations of intervention withdrawal being achieved. For example, Heyman (1987) managed to get an amateur boxer to cease using a hypnotic intervention that was successful in silencing the sound of the crowd. The boxer found the sound of the crowd anxiety-inducing and detrimental to performance. The boxer was very pleased with the success of the intervention but agreed not to use the intervention in one fight only before it was re-introduced.

In single-case research, by using an A–B–A–B design it is possible to demonstrate the replicability of effects (Kratochwill et al. 1984). In an A–B–A–B design, this can be done by observing changes in the dependent (target) variables following the introduction, removal and re-introduction of the intervention. It is also possible to observe if similar changes occur across participants using a multiple-baseline design. This involves collecting baseline and post-intervention data across several individuals. The validity of the intervention is determined by observing changes in the target variable(s) after introducing the intervention. If similar changes are observed across participants it supports the efficacy of the technique employed. To illustrate, an exercise psychologist may be working with three factory workers to increase adherence to a daily workout session run by their employers. To increase attendance, the psychologist introduces a time management intervention a fortnight apart for each exerciser. If the time management intervention is successful, attendance should increase for each exerciser when the intervention is introduced. There are many examples of multiple-baseline studies in sport and exercise (see Chapters 2 and 6).

In summary, different designs in single-case research use similar elements to the group designs common to sport and exercise research. Despite this range of designs the validity of single-case research as a scientific endeavour has been questioned and this is considered in more detail in Chapter 2, in which the principles of scientific research are outlined. We now turn to consider why single-case research designs are useful in sport and exercise.

Why are single-case research designs useful?

We do not propose that single-case research designs should replace controlled group designs. There are many questions (e.g., 'Which of two different interventions works best for a group of athletes?') that are best answered using group designs. So, single-case research designs and group designs can be complementary. Instead, a key theme of this book is that single-case research can be a useful addition to a range of research methodologies. Coaches, sport and exercise psychologists, sport and exercise physiologists, and biomechanists draw upon many strategies and interventions to produce targeted changes in athletes' or exercisers' thoughts, emotions, behaviour, physical states, techniques or performances. This work is often done at an individual level. Accordingly, it makes sense that the efficacy of the interventions used is *demonstrated* at an individual level. For example, many sport psychologists use imagery as a psychological skill when working with athletes, yet the most frequently cited evidence for its effectiveness comes from group studies in which the imagery technique may be taught and delivered in a different way from that used between a consultant and client. In group-based designs treatments are typically administered and behaviour assessed in a more contrived and controlled laboratory environment (Kazdin 1982). Moreover, findings from a group study may mask individual differences in responding to the intervention, and in an applied setting a practitioner is seldom concerned with bringing about a statistically significant change in group averages but rather with making meaningful changes at an individual level. In short, the efficacy of an intervention should be demonstrated in the situation in which it is to be deployed, and single-case research promotes naturalistic applied settings to assess and observe participants after interventions have been applied (Kazdin 1982). Naturalistic settings also encourage treatment effects to be observed on ecologically valid tasks (e.g., actual sport performance). This provides researchers with further information about the efficacy of techniques along with their application and integration in actual sport and exercise situations. In sum, single-case research can take place in naturalistic settings and be ecologically valid.

The value of single-case research in determining the effectiveness of interventions can be illustrated if a distinction is made between evaluation *research* and evaluation of *practice* (see Anderson, Miles, Mahoney and Robinson 2002). To explain, evaluation research involves testing a particular intervention in a controlled environment whereas the evaluation of practice involves investigating the outcome of an intervention as it would actually be delivered (Seligman 1995). It is in this latter approach that single-case research has a clear role to play.

Single-case research can usefully determine the effectiveness of interventions and add value to the controlled group research that is typical of much of the research in sport and exercise. In a controlled group design a group that receives an intervention is typically compared on performance and other dependent variables with a control group. However, the validity of relying solely on such an approach to determine the effectiveness of psychological skills interventions has been questioned and, as a result, researchers have been encouraged to use single-case research designs where appropriate (see Hrycaiko and Martin 1996; Mace 1990). A major benefit of single-case research is that it enables the practitioner to provide individualized, as opposed to standardized, training. This advantage is especially relevant when one considers that in studies using controlled group designs, although the overall results may show no difference, it is possible that the treatment worked for some individuals (Mace 1990). This is more than simply an issue of statistical power. It is a recognition that individuals may differ in their preference and ability to use different interventions. As controlled studies should consist of homogeneous groups it could be argued that this problem should not apply. However, it is often difficult to obtain large numbers of participants who are homogeneous on all relevant characteristics, particularly skill level. This has resulted in many controlled studies consisting of novice participants (e.g., Mace and Carroll 1985) and there is an obvious limitation in generalizing results gained from novice participants to more experienced, skilful performers. Large group studies with elite performers rarely happen because of the difficulties of getting large numbers of participants. For example, if a researcher wished to explore the effectiveness of biofeedback as an anxiety control strategy in high-level archers, it would be impossible, first, to get a large number of Olympic archers with a similar level of anxiety and, second, to get them all to agree to participate in a study. In short, single-case research provides the opportunity to explore the efficacy of techniques in unique or uncommon populations.

From a research perspective, a controlled study with performers may mask any small but consistent improvements in performance that have practical significance for the athlete (Bryan 1987). This may be particularly crucial for elite athletes for whom even small improvements in performance may result in substantial changes in outcome. It may also mask individual differences in the responses to the interventions. As Morgan and Morgan (2001, p. 125) noted:

> group designs intended to identify effective interventions necessarily produce 'conditional' knowledge, in that treatment efficacy will ultimately depend on several separate factors, some of which pertain to idiosyncratic client features. These idiosyncratic features, ordinarily beyond the scope of a large group study, are the heart and soul of single-participant designs.

Briefly, a single-case research design can not only identify whether or not a particular intervention is effective but also illuminate how effective it is with what type of participants. Single-case research can also provide evidence about how interventions should be delivered along with examples of good practice.

Why are single-case research designs important for both researcher and practitioner?

Much of the applied work in sport and exercise (see Hemmings and Holder 2009) is conducted with small samples or individuals and it makes sense to determine change in small samples or individuals. Indeed, finding methods to rigorously determine change along with consultant and/or coach effectiveness are important issues for the sport and exercise community and stakeholders. Single-case research can provide evidence for the effectiveness of interventions, and this is important for researchers and practitioners as this type of information is beneficial to the marketing of sport and exercise services as well as identifying individual differences in treatment efficacy (Hrycaiko and Martin 1996).

Evaluating intervention work is important for practitioners and this is best achieved through the use of rigorous single-case research designs. In this regard,

Anderson et al. (2002) have outlined why sport psychologists should evaluate their services (although this is applicable to other sport and exercise practitioners). First, the sport psychologist has an ethical responsibility to the athlete and/or secondary clients such as the coach or governing body to monitor and evaluate the support offered. Second, sport psychologists are accountable to themselves and should continue to strive to improve effectiveness and provide the best possible service. Evaluating the work done is a key part of this. Third, and more broadly, sport psychologists are accountable to the profession and must be able to demonstrate effectiveness to the appropriate professional bodies. The evaluation of interventions can help demonstrate knowledge and, although Anderson et al. did not consider this a primary reason for evaluation, it is important to increase the credibility of the field. In short, demonstrating effectiveness is of equal importance to both researchers and practitioners.

Summary

Single-case research designs are a common feature in behavioural and health sciences settings with a number of excellent publications guiding work in this area (e.g., Barlow, Nock and Hersen 2009; Kazdin 1982; Morgan and Morgan 2009). Yet the use and dissemination of single-case research into the sport and exercise literature has been less prevalent, which is surprising given the applied nature of sport and exercise science disciplines (Kinugasa, Cerin and Hooper 2004). Choosing a single-case approach is valuable, particularly when embarking on new research areas. Single-case designs allow the detection of positive effects for individuals who would otherwise have their success masked in a non-significant group design. Furthermore, single-case research designs allow programmes to be tailored for individuals engaged in real-life sport. Finally, single-case research has the potential to demonstrate to consumers of sport and exercise services that improvements in athletic and exercise performance are due to interventions.

Single-case research remains somewhat underused in sport and exercise in comparison with the behavioural and health domains. Perhaps this reflects a lack of acceptance and reluctance by researchers and practitioners (Hrycaiko and Martin 1996). Although the publication of studies involving single-case designs within sport and exercise is increasing (e.g., Barker and Jones 2006, 2008; Kinugasa et al. 2004; McCarthy, Jones, Harwood and Davenport 2010) many practitioners within the area do not understand how best to apply the single-case method. Perhaps this is exacerbated by an irregular coverage of single-case research methods within many undergraduate and postgraduate sport and exercise science degree programmes.

The purpose of this book is to review single-case research in sport and exercise and introduce the philosophical and procedural features of single-case research. It is intended for students, researchers and practitioners. Single-case research represents an effective (yet currently underused) complement to group research allowing researchers and consultants to determine the efficacy of biomechanical, physiological, psychological and coaching-related interventions in the applied setting of the sports field or exercise room. The remaining chapters will present the philosophical and historical development, design procedures and features, analysis strategies and contemporary use of single-case research methods in sport and exercise.

Key points

- The use of single-case research designs in sport and exercise can help increase knowledge.
- In case studies, observations are made under uncontrolled and unsystematic conditions.
- In a single-case research design it is possible to have control over the independent variables in a manner similar to that observed in group designs.
- Single-case research designs can provide a scientific approach to understanding the effectiveness of interventions in sport and exercise settings.
- Evaluating intervention work using single-case research designs is important for both researchers and practitioners and is beneficial to the sport and exercise science discipline.

Guided study

Your first task is to locate a study that used a single-case research design from an academic journal in sport and exercise. For example, you might examine *The Sport Psychologist, Psychology of Sport and Exercise* or the *Journal of Applied Sport Psychology*. Once you have located your journal article you should read it and answer the following questions:

- Which topic, from a sport and exercise context, is under examination?
- Which example of single-case research design is the author is using?
- What were the outcomes from the study?
- How does the paper contribute to the literature?
- What limitations did the author expose?
- What limitations do you notice?
- What are the particular strengths of the paper?

2

HISTORY AND PHILOSOPHY OF SINGLE-CASE RESEARCH IN SPORT AND EXERCISE

In this chapter, we will:

- outline the development of the scientific method;
- summarize the background to single-case research in psychology;
- examine the development of single-case research in sport and exercise.

Introduction

Many research methods modules in sport and exercise either do not include single-case research designs or else refer to them fleetingly – explaining that they are potentially useful for sport and exercise practitioners engaged in research and practice. A possible reason for this neglect of single-case research designs is that those who teach research methods to undergraduates and postgraduates are committed to the principles and practices of group design research (Hrycaiko and Martin 1996). Indeed, with a strong emphasis on group design research, the salient features of single-case designs often remain outside students', practitioners' and researchers' repertoire of research skills in sport and exercise. This lack of attention towards single-case research seems strange for at least three reasons. First, many practitioners (e.g., sport psychologists and exercise physiologists) consult with only one or just a few athletes at a time and so they need a research method that is suitable to understand behaviour change among these clients (Kinugasa et al. 2004). This is an important element of evaluating practice (Seligman 1995), outlined in Chapter 1. Second, specific issues such as injury or burnout cannot always be studied using group designs because recruiting sufficiently large numbers to conduct meaningful research is impractical (Kinugasa et al. 2004). Finally, from a historical perspective, many classic findings have come from research using single-case designs (Mook 2001). We have already outlined the work of Ebbinghaus on memory in Chapter 1. In addition, over 100 years ago, the famous Russian physiologist and learning theorist, Ivan Pavlov, conducted many experiments that involved one or only a few participants (i.e., 'small *n*' research). In his experiments on classical conditioning, Pavlov presented a stimulus that evoked an unconditioned response (e.g., food in the dog's mouth evoked salivation). He paired the stimulus with another conditioned stimulus (e.g., the sound of a bell ringing) that did not evoke the response initially. After conditioning, however, the conditioned stimulus evoked the response. In other words, the ringing of a bell made the dog salivate. One of the most influential papers in the history of American psychology (Miller 1960) emerged from Watson and Rayner's (1920) study of Albert, whom they conditioned to fear a white rat. This study appeared to support the notion that conditioning could establish enduring traits of personality such as our emotional tendencies (Dukes 1965; Murphy 1949). These designs have offered, and continue to offer, a useful method to examine the behaviour of a single case (i.e., one subject) in a natural or experimental setting (Kazdin 1982). Yet the potted history of science and research design we present next suggests that single-case design research represents a radical departure from traditional research. In this chapter we shall briefly explain early scientific inquiry and provide a historical context for the basic principles of the scientific method outlined in Chapter 1. Then we shall explore the history of experimental designs before presenting the history and philosophy of single-case research in sport and exercise.

Early scientific inquiry

Many individuals and movements throughout history weaved the fabric of science as we study it today. Each contribution aimed to advance our control of performance variables and to model behavioural phenomena mathematically (Ittenbach and Lawhead 1996). Primarily, researchers and practitioners are concerned with measurement; yet this concern has a long history that shaped the research design we now study. For instance, in 585 BC, Thales, a Greek thinker, predicted a solar eclipse after making careful observations of the heavens. Rather than accepting such events as the will of the gods, he noticed that they emerged from a consistent, natural order that could be studied, generalized and predicted. The Pythagoreans, for example, believed that all things could be understood by numbers, and Pythagoras' theorem offers an enduring example of their influence. Anaximenes (c. 545 BC) is credited with the first scientific experiment in recorded history. Specifically he reported that changing the shape of one's mouth produced changes in the temperature of the air one exhaled. In other words, he established that 'quantitative changes in performance produced qualitative changes in an event' (Ittenbach and Lawhead 1996, p. 16).

Readers are perhaps more familiar with the following Greek thinkers who not only established the basics for contemporary scientific inquiry but also each contributed to the development of philosophical ideas that continue to influence

Western thought: Socrates (c. 470–399 BC), Plato (c. 428–348 BC) and Aristotle (c. 384–322 BC). Although Socrates left no written records of his ideas, his thoughts and ideas have come through in the writings of other scholars such as Plato and Aristotle. Socrates believed in fixed and stable truths, unlike his immediate philosophical predecessors, the Sophists, who believed it was impossible for people to know anything. But this knowledge was only possible through introspective and disciplined inquiry. Only through discussion and rigorous questioning could some idea become knowledge or a stable truth. Today we refer to this as the Socratic (or dialectic) method (Ittenbach and Lawhead 1996). It comprises a sequence of repetitions in which an initial opinion is criticized, modified and criticized again, until a stable truth emerges. And it is precisely this method that is also exercised by sport psychologists in professional practice today. Socratic dialogue represents one technique practised by sport psychologists to change cognitions and establish appropriate emotional responses (Jones 2003). This technique involves the sport psychologist asking thought-provoking questions to persuade the athlete to re-evaluate self-defeating ideas and misperceptions.

Plato, a student of Socrates, established an integrated system of reasoning to join distinct areas of thought (e.g., politics, ethics, physics). He believed in scientific inquiry and acknowledged that mathematical reasoning could reveal the reality of all things. Plato also suggested that human personality could be divided into three parts: reason, spirit and appetites. Each person has these three faculties; however, one will dominate in each individual. Aristotle modified the contributions of Socrates and Plato, classifying science into theoretical and practical sciences. Theoretical science represented the pursuit of knowledge for its own sake whereas practical science involved knowledge that could be used to alter the course of events. This division reflects our current distinction between basic and applied research. For example, basic research might involve testing a hypothesis related to achievment goal theory (Nicholls 1984, 1989) whereas applied research might use the tenets of this theory to solve a practical problem such as motivating students to continue participating in physical education.

Traditions of experimental design

Until the thirteenth and fourteenth centuries, intellectual life focused mainly on theology and so the need to explore aspects of the world scientifically was not demanded. From the fifteenth to the nineteenth centuries, however, critical advances through experimentation allowed specific research fields to develop, such as electromagnetism and the study of gases and mechanics. We can trace the evolution of mechanics from Galileo though Newton to Einstein along with many other fields of study. When we examine these fields of inquiry, we notice that controlled conditions allowed researchers to permit a single observation at a time. Observations were repeated to ensure repeatability and to draw comparisons with their first observations. Scientists experiment to expose empirical comparisons when naturalistic observation alone is inadequate (Johnston and

Pennypacker 1993). The experiment comprises conditions designed to gain information which supports a conclusion that would not be possible without such conditions. You read this text from a privileged perspective because you know more about experimental designs than many of the early researchers. For instance, sample sizes, control groups and data evaluation using statistical analysis became popular only with the advent of statistical methods. Much of the early research in sport psychology studies (e.g., Triplett 1898) did not use inferential statistics because they had not been invented at that stage. These methods allowed researchers to establish group differences and similarities.

Experimental design, as we know it today, involves many methods of varying complexity. For instance, it depends heavily on inferential statistics. But where did statistics begin? Walker (1929) studied the history of statistical method and identified three traditions that underlie scientific inference based on group comparisons: social enumeration, economic quantification and mathematical statistics. Social enumeration refers to people and property, amongst other things, that we count. In England, for instance, the *Domesday Book* listed the landowners and an inventory of their property. Economic quantification allowed monarchs to quantify people and resources to equip them for military pursuits. And mathematical statistics developed the mathematics of probability amongst others. Johnston and Pennypacker (1993) suggested a fourth dimension to add to the three identified by Walker, that of agricultural experimentation.

Three people are intricately involved in the evolution of the statistical method for designing experiments: Francis Galton, Karl Pearson and Ronald Fisher. Francis Galton (1822–1911) involved himself in education, especially mental measurement, which continues as a research field in psychology today. Galton was fascinated with variation within and between measures, which led him to develop the first mathematical expression of correlation. Karl Pearson (1857–1936) developed Galton's proposal and Edgeworth developed the first correlation coefficient in 1892. Pearson introduced the term standard deviation and the mathematics of sampling distributions. Finally, Ronald Fisher, a trained mathematician and biologist, was intensely interested in evolution and heredity but turned his focus to agriculture. Fisher and his colleagues developed statistical methods to evaluate agricultural data and he published *The Design of Experiments* in 1935 (Fisher 1935). Single-case research designs had small sample sizes and an absence of controls that displeased researchers (Chaddock 1925). The publication of Fisher's book on statistics (Fisher 1925) resulted in a major change in how researchers conducted experiments. This book emphasized the significance of comparing groups of subjects and presented the structures underlying the analyses of variance test. Journal publications in the 1930s reflected the move from small sample studies with no statistical evaluation to larger sample studies with statistical evaluation (Boring 1954). Although researchers and journals reported single-case investigations, journals published much less of them than before. Next came the dominance of the basic control group design and it became the paradigm of psychological research. In this design, the researcher gives the experimental group(s) the treatment but withholds treatment from the control group and assesses the differences between the groups. Statistical methods are used to decide the statistical differences between the groups based on levels of confidence (probability levels) selected before the study (Kazdin 1982).

Fisher's work, and that of his colleagues, focused on descriptions of population characteristics using means and standard deviations. When we consider measurement in sport and exercise, especially large-scale evaluation, the researcher is concerned with a particular procedure and its effect on the sample (or more precisely the population from which that sample is drawn) rather than on a particular athlete. Johnston and Pennypacker (1993) explained that the generality of group comparisons to the individual case is problematic because behaviour is a phenomenon that occurs at the individual level. Psychology, as the science of behaviour, however, must attempt to understand the individual and his or her interaction with the environment. When we achieve this process, then we can address the question of generalizing the results from one or a few individuals to a larger population. McNemar (1940, p. 361) asserted that:

> The statistician who fails to see that important generalizations from research on a single case can ever be acceptable is on a par with the experimentalist who fails to appreciate the fact that some problems can never be solved without resort to numbers.

In short, single-case research can make a contribution. We now turn to consider whether single-case research designs can be scientific. A criticism of single-case research is that it is unscientific because of its use of small numbers and because of the absence of comparison or control groups (see Jones 1996). To counter this criticism, we explore the purpose of research and whether research conducted using a single-case research design can be scientific.

Research is usually seen as having at least one of four aims: to describe, understand, predict and control (Clark-Carter 2009). To illustrate, we shall consider the influence of anxiety on sport performance. A researcher may seek to describe the symptoms of anxiety (e.g., racing heart, worry); understand how symptoms of anxiety arise and how it influences cognitive and physical functioning; predict how these symptoms influence performance; or explore the efficacy of techniques to control anxiety levels in competition. It is possible for single-case research to address all of these aims. But most studies in this field address the fourth aim (namely, to achieve experimental control), with most single-case research papers exploring the efficacy of an intervention.

To consider whether single-case research addressing one or more of these aims is scientific, it is important to define the basic principles of a scientific method. Broadly, there are two contrasting approaches to the scientific method: positivism and postpositivism (falsification). Positivism (or the theory that empirical science provides the only valid form of knowledge; see Tolman 1991) emerged out of the modernist era through the writings of philosophers such as Auguste Comte, John Stuart Mill and David Hume (Brustad 2002). According to this perspective, the natural world follows systematic, orderly and predictable laws that humans are considered capable of understanding and shaping to their benefit (Gergen 1991). Scientific research involves the study of that which is measurable, quantifiable, objectifiable and observable with human senses. A researcher will develop a testable statement (e.g., music during an exercise class will increase participants' work rates), which will be tested through empirical means.

However, critics of positivism, such as the philosopher Karl Popper, have argued that this approach encourages researchers to be more concerned with justifying a theory rather than running the risk of falsifying it with counterevidence (Gregory 2004). Accordingly, falsifiability is a better criterion for any theory and researchers should be encouraged to generate hypotheses. All good hypotheses should be falsifiable and, in light of the evidence collected, hypotheses are supported, abandoned or modified, although Popper preferred that hypotheses be accepted or rejected as one that could be modified in the light of the evidence was one that had not been phrased correctly to be sufficiently falsifiable in the first place (Gregory 2004).

The positivist approach requires researchers to develop statements that can be tested and proven while postpositivists require researchers to develop hypotheses that are falsifiable. This may seem a pedantic distinction but the approach adopted does reflect our understanding of whether we actually truly know anything or whether we will have a set of hypotheses that have simply yet to be disproven. In a sense, postpositivists have a more limited view of our ability to really 'know' than positivists (Brustad 2002). It is not possible to determine that one explanation is correct because it is not possible to test all competing theories. However, scientists can have confidence in their theories by ruling out plausible alternative explanations and as this cannot be achieved in a single study it illustrates why science is a cumulative process (Conroy, Kaye and Schantz 2002).

We have outlined two contrasting approaches to scientific research (for a more detailed discussion see Brustad 2002 and Conroy et al. 2002). Although it is a broad overview of what constitutes scientific research, it should be apparent that single-case research should be able to *either* test propositions *or* falsify hypotheses. One way of testing propositions or of falsifying hypotheses is by having sufficient control in the design, that is, control over the independent variables and extraneous variables that may influence the data. Perhaps the biggest challenge in single-case research is having control over the extraneous variables given that much of the research is conducted in the field. For example, a psychologist may be working with a basketball player who is lacking in confidence and data are collected for a baseline phase, but the basketball player is dropped from the starting team before the intervention can begin so all follow-up data are collected from the less-demanding second-team environment. Clearly such a situation poses not only methodological but also ethical challenges for researchers. Despite these challenges, sufficient control over key target variables can be achieved using single-case designs – thereby enabling valid and meaningful conclusions to be drawn from the data collected. We now turn to expand on the differences between case studies and single-case research and expand on the issues touched upon in Chapter 1.

Case studies and single-case research

We have already outlined in Chapter 1 examples of uncontrolled case studies. Such studies did not interest serious applied researchers in the 1940s and 1950s because it was difficult to appraise the effects of the treatment (Barlow et al. 2009). At this time, clinicians (e.g., psychiatrists) lacked the necessary equipment for collecting data during the therapeutic hour. They were reluctant to collect detailed notes and were concerned about confidentiality. But clinicians believed that the case-study method could be useful in generating new hypotheses that could be tested more rigorously in subsequent experiments (Barlow et al. 2009). Many scientists and clinicians were unable to distinguish between the *uncontrolled* case study and the *experimental* study of an individual. This problem impeded the theoretical development and practical implementation of single-case experimental designs. In the next section, we build on the material covered in Chapter 1 by expanding on the characteristics of the case study and outline how reseachers and practitioners distinguish it from single-case experimental designs.

According to Stake (2000, p. 436), a case study is 'both a process of inquiry about the case and the product of that inquiry' – especially when the inquiry is 'specific, unique, and bounded'. The case study presents a common method of conducting qualitative inquiry in various branches of psychology. Indeed, one could argue that most studies published in sport and exercise psychology journals are influenced more by researchers' interest in individual cases than in the methods used. In other words, the methods organize the case for the practitioner but rarely drive the process. Case studies vary in complexity, with some studies involving a single case such as a psychologist testing an individual who is unique in some theoretically interesting way (Smith 1988; Stake 1988). For instance, Krane, Greenleaf and Snow (1997) presented a qualitative case study of a former elite gymnast using the social-cognitive approach to achievement motivation to understand and explain the behaviour of the gymnast, her coaches and her parents. Sometimes researchers and practitioners overlook the distinction between single-case research designs and case studies (Blampied 2000). Case studies are usually descriptive and normally cannot support valid causal inferences whereas experimental single-case research attempts to reject the null hypothesis (Sidman 1960); emphasizes visual analysis of data in graphs (Parsonson and Baer 1978, 1992; see also Chapter 9); and relies on replication to make reliable causal inferences (Sidman 1960). Single-case research designs are controlled experiments from which to draw causal inferences (Sidman 1960) but, as we explained at the beginning of this chapter, they are a neglected alternative in standard textbooks on research methods (Blampied 2000).

Background of single-case research

Gordon Allport (1937, 1962) described the study of broad, general, universal laws, and the methods used in such study, as nomothetic, from the Greek word *nomos*, meaning law; and the study of individuals and the methods involved in this field of study as idiographic, from the Greek word *idios*, meaning one's own or private experience. Psychoanalysis, for example, both as a theory of personality and as a treatment technique developed from a relatively small number of cases seen by Freud (1933–1964) in outpatient psychotherapy. He developed his theory of psychoanalysis from this intense study of the individual. Psychotherapy techniques have benefited most from the study of individual cases. Well-known cases throughout the history of clinical work have stimulated major developments in theory and practice. Studying the individual case aided many disciplines of psychology. For instance, our understanding of the brain and its functions has been greatly helped by intensive studies of individuals such as Phineas Gage, whom you read about in Chapter 1. Burrhus Frederic Skinner and his colleagues refined the single-case method in their study of animal behaviour to develop a sophisticated methodology allowing researchers and practitioners to study individual cases intensively (Barlow et al. 2009). The publication of Sidman's (1960) *Tactics of Scientific Research* marked the definitive methodology of single-case research, explaining the assumptions and conditions of a true experimental analysis of behaviour. Skinner and his colleagues established the *Journal of Experimental Analysis of Behavior* (*JEAB*) in 1958 to overcome the reluctance of editors of major psychological journals to publish their work using data from single subjects (Morgan and Morgan 2009). The experimental study of the single case in basic and applied research was marked with a journal in 1968 (*Journal of Applied Behavior Analysis*). The experimental study of the single case then appeared in major psychological and psychiatric journals. Basic research methodology was termed experimental analysis of behaviour and applied problems were termed *behaviour modification* or *behaviour therapy* (Barlow et al. 2009).

A brief history of single-case research in sport and exercise

Sport and exercise psychology represents a relatively young discipline in psychology. But it would be remiss of us to overlook that many researchers were interested in the psychological influences on sport behaviour shortly after the emergence of psychology in the late nineteenth century. In particular, Norman Triplett was intrigued by the popular knowlege of that time suggesting that racing cyclists go faster when racing, or when paced, than when riding alone (Hogg and Vaughan 2008; Kremer and Moran 2008). His most famous experiment involved schoolchildren working in two conditions, alone and in pairs. They used fishing reels that turned silk bands around a drum. Many social psychologists regard this experiment as the first experimental study in social psychology but sport psychologists have claimed this study as their own (Vaughan and Guerin 1997). In the early part of the twentieth century, an educational psychologist, Coleman R. Griffith, began writing, researching and practising sport psychology. He also contributed two books to the discipline: *The Psychology of Coaching* (Griffith 1926) and *Psychology of Athletics* (Griffith 1928). But it was much later in the twentieth century before applied sport psychology developed in earnest.

In 1972, Rushall and Siedentop first described behavioural applications in sports in their book *The Development and Control of Behavior in Sport and Physical Education* (Rushall and Siedentop 1972). This book drew heavily from Skinner's writings and outlined practical strategies to shape new sport skills and generalize practice skills to competitive settings (Martin, Thompson and Regehr 2004). In 1974, the *Journal of Applied Behavior Analysis* published the first research in applied behaviour analysis in a sport setting. The authors, McKenzie and Rushall, examined the effects of self-recording on attendance and performance in a competitive swimming training environment. Other substantial contributions to behavioural sport psychology emerged in the 1970s, especially the work of Smith, Smoll and their colleagues, who examined the effects of assessment and modification of behaviours of Little League baseball coaches (Smith, Smoll and Hunt 1977; Smith, Smoll and Curtis 1979). Single-case designs by Allison and Ayllon (1980) used behavioural coaching to develop skills in football, gymnastics and tennis, and Koop and Martin (1983) also evaluated a coaching strategy to reduce swimming stroke errors in beginning age-group swimmers.

In the late 1970s to early 1990s, several journals were established (e.g., *Journal of Sport Behavior* in 1979; *Journal of Sport Psychology* in 1979, renamed the *Journal of Sport & Exercise Psychology* in 1988; *The Sport Psychologist* in 1987; and the *Journal of Applied Sport Psychology* in 1989), numerous books were published and the frequency of national and international conferences increased. Since McKenzie and Rushall's (1974) study in applied behaviour analysis, there has been a steady increase in single-case designs in sport and exercise over the past thirty-five years. However, although single-case research designs form a significant and useful tool to examine behaviour change and intervention effects in sport and exercise contexts, this method has largely been neglected by researchers in these areas (Hrycaiko and Martin 1996). This trend is changing, but the change is slow. Hrycaiko and Martin established that only twelve articles using single-case designs emerged from the three major sport psychology journals up to 1994: *Journal of Sport & Exercise Psychology*, *The Sport Psychologist* and the *Journal of Applied Sport Psychology*. Since 1994, many more studies using single-case designs have emerged, and journals such as the *Psychology of Sport and Exercise* ($n = 7$) and the *Sport and Exercise Psychology Review* ($n = 4$) among others have contributed to that increase.

The lack of studies using single-case designs is surprising because these designs can neatly examine the applied work of sport and exercise psychologists in professional practice. More recently, Martin et al. (2004) examined single-case design studies published in sport psychology journals and behavioural journals between 1974 and 2004. Each decade witnessed a steady increase in single-case designs, from 0.6 published articles each year to 1.2 and 2.2 during the past three decades, respectively. Hrycaiko and Martin (1996) suggested a few reasons why so few single-case designs are published in sport and exercise psychology journals. First, research funding agencies appear to favour group designs over single-case designs, perhaps because of the traditional dominance of the nomothetic approach and the medical model in research in psychology. It might also be the case that students and supervisors do not understand the single-case designs. This misunderstanding might have arisen because single-case designs are rarely, if ever, taught in university programmes. Quantitative research methods dominate the modules on research methods with much less attention paid to qualitative or single-case research designs. But as we argue throughout this book, single-case designs have much to offer researchers and practitioners in sport and exercise. To begin with, in 1966, Abraham Maslow wrote 'by far the best way we have to learn what people are like is to get them . . . to tell us about themselves' (Maslow 1966, p. 12). When sport psychologists consult with sport performers, they engage in dialogue to establish a route for their consultation. For example, they might identify one or more target behaviour(s) to address and measure during a baseline phase. Then the sport psychologist might implement a treatment whilst continuing to measure the target behaviour(s) throughout the treatment phase. Sport psychologists often use single-case designs to provide evidence-based interventions for use in applied work with sport performers. Not surprisingly, therefore, many sport psychologists use single-case designs to justify the strength of their applied work with sport performers (Smith 1988; Hemmings and Holder 2009). Indeed to advance applied sport psychology, sport psychologists need experimental, quasi-experimental and non-experimental research methods. An experimental approach to evaluation might include randomized control group, quasi-experimental or single-participant designs to show that only the intervention caused the change. This experimental approach ensures that the design has high internal validity (an aspect of research designs we shall explore in Chapter 9), but in professional practice this design is impractical, especially when you offer a service to one group of athletes and deliberately withhold that service from another group of athletes (Anderson et al. 2002). If the needs of one athlete are the only ones in question, then single-participant designs are practitioner-friendly in practical settings, despite these designs being time-consuming and expensive (Anderson et al. 2002; Barlow, Hayes and Nelson 1984; Smith 1988).

Summary

Most students of sport and exercise receive more teaching about group designs than about single-case research in research methods courses. Students recognize the characteristics of group designs; for example, researchers group participants, usually present data as group averages and calculate the reliability of differences among conditions by a test of statistical significance (Mook 2001). The opposite is true for single-case designs. The researcher treats each participant as a separate experiment and examines differences among conditions in each participant's data. Individual participants' data are presented and reliability is tested by replication. In this chapter we have provided a historical context for single-case research and outlined how single-case research designs have an important role in sport and exercise for researchers and practitioners. Single-case designs have scientific rigour and, in the following chapters, we shall explain how to conduct valuable research using this design.

Key points

- Science has a long history and individuals as well as movements shaped the research methods we use today.
- Many significant findings in the early development of psychology began with the study of a single case.
- Researchers dissatisfied with the measurement rigour of a case study favoured group designs, which have dominated basic and applied research to this day.
- The past forty years have witnessed an increase in single-case research designs in sport and exercise and this research method contributes to the healthy development of research and applied practice in sport and exercise.

Guided study

Your task in this chapter is to locate two studies from sport and exercise psychology journals, one that uses a single-case research design and one that uses a group design. You'll find examples in the *Journal of Applied Behavioral Analysis*, *The Sport Psychologist*, *Psychology of Sport and Exercise* and the *Journal of Applied Sport Psychology*. For each study, explain:

- What similarities and differences emerge between the samples used?
- Which type of design is used?
- Which type of analysis is used?
- What were the limitations of each paper?
- Whether you believe the research method used was appropriate for the topic under examination.

3

GENERAL PROCEDURES IN SINGLE-CASE RESEARCH

In this chapter, we will outline issues to consider in:

* the planning of single-case research;
* the conduct of single case-research;
* the interpretation of data in single-case research.

Introduction

In this chapter we consider examples of good practice that enhance the rigour of single-case research and we also outline issues that help critical consideration of the data collected. By reflecting regularly and critically on our research and practice we can identify occasions in which we have come up a little short of the standards required. This activity is the key to being an effective reflective practitioner in any professional field. To begin the chapter, we consider issues in collecting data, the type of data that can be collected and how meaningful change can be determined in single-case research. We then consider issues surrounding variability in the data, including different types of baseline, and we conclude by describing what should be considered when presenting data graphically.

Data collection

It is obvious that the strength of a single-case research paper will depend on the quality of the data collected. There are at least four ways in which data can be collected: by interview, self-report measures (including psychometric tests), observation and physiological testing. We do not discuss the strengths, weaknesses and good practice of different assessment techniques in sport and exercise settings as these are beyond the scope of the present book. For a good coverage of these issues, the reader is directed to such sources as Duda (1998), Gardner and Moore (2006) and Thomas, Nelson and Silverman (2005). Instead, we begin this chapter by focusing on three issues that relate to data collection in single-case research. First, we consider the role of the assessment phase before outlining the importance of clearly defining the behaviour or target variable to be observed and describing the Hawthorne effect.

The assessment phase

Most single-case research involves determining the utility of an intervention designed to bring about a meaningful change to a participant. In these situations, a participant may present themselves to a researcher with an issue to resolve. Before collecting baseline data the researcher needs to decide what the baseline data will consist of, and this is done during the assessment phase. For example, if a field hockey player reports that worries and physical tension are impairing her performance then the researcher might use a standardized psychometric instrument such as the Competitive State Anxiety Inventory-2 (CSAI-2; Martens, Burton, Vealey, Bump and Smith 1990) to collect baseline data. The baseline phase is then the period in which the variables of interest identified in the assessment phase are monitored. The assessment phase is crucial because it helps the researcher understand the problem and guides the format of the baseline phase.

A frequently used approach in single-case research is to interview the participant (see Yukelson 2010 for guidelines on effective interviewing). Of particular interest in the context of single-case research is deciding *who* to interview. It may strengthen the research to interview people close to the participant, and if this is possible it helps the researcher to get a different perspective on the issue to be addressed. For example, to understand a young mother's difficulties in adhering to an exercise programme it may be helpful to interview her partner and other family members about her approach to exercise and the barriers that exist, and she may be happy for this to happen. However, on occasion it may not be practical or ethical to interview people other than the participant. To illustrate, a professional soccer player may contact a psychologist because of difficulty dealing with the stress of important matches and the psychologist may wish to gather information from the player's manager and other members of the coaching staff. But it is quite possible that the player would be uncomfortable with other individuals being interviewed, and the researcher for reasons of confidentiality will be unable to conduct the interviews. In short, although the research, and the development of the intervention, would benefit from a number of interviews being conducted, it may not be ethical to do so and priority should be given to the professional codes of practice to which the researcher adheres. This is an illustration of a common theme in single-case research in applied settings of the tension between the strongest possible research design and the demands of working that may not always allow this to happen. Interviewing is only one way of collecting data during an assessment phase and similar issues may arise with the use of other assessment techniques.

Regardless of the assessment techniques used it is important to collect sufficient data to provide an accurate picture of the issue to be addressed. Collecting data using complementary methods can help, and triangulation of data will outline a more complete picture of the issue to be addressed, whereas relying on one measure may leave a researcher developing an intervention that is unsuitable. To illustrate, one of us (Jones) began working with a young hockey player who reported debilitating levels of anxiety during matches and felt he was being unfairly criticized by his teammates for errors during these matches. Data were collected from interviews with the participant and the CSAI-2 (Martens et al. 1990) was revised to assess perceptions of anxiety symptoms (Jones and Swain 1992), completed over seven games. The participant did indeed report debilitating and high levels of competitive anxiety and an intervention was developed to help him deal with his anxiety that comprised imagery of successful past performances before matches and positive self-talk to deal with the criticism from his teammates. The participant, however, had not been observed in competition and during informal conversations with his teammates (unrelated to the intervention) it transpired that the participant himself was very critical of his teammates. Perhaps not surprisingly, because he had been very critical of his fellow teammates, when he himself made a mistake his teammates would take the opportunity to point this out vociferously. A large part of the intervention should have focused on developing more suitable ways for the participant to interact with his teammates but because the assessment phase was inadequate this was not addressed and this aspect of his behaviour was not monitored.

Observation

The preceding example clearly illustrates the importance of observation and how it can be an essential part of the assessment phase, and also, as we shall discuss later in this chapter, that monitoring and changing behaviour is probably the most important element in sport and exercise. We outline in more detail in Chapter 4 how behavioural assessment can best take place. There are also some clear guidelines provided for single-case (Morgan and Morgan 2009) and sport and exercise (Gardner and Moore 2006; Thomas et al. 2005) researchers. In this chapter we begin the focus on behavioural assessment by looking at two key issues outlined by Morgan and Morgan (2009) that are relevant to observation in sport and exercise.

First, Morgan and Morgan (2009) outlined the importance of defining the behaviour (or target behaviour) to be observed and why it is crucial to be clear how this behaviour will be observed and measured. These researchers use the example of aggression to illustrate the importance of defining the behaviour to be observed and this example is also particularly applicable to sport settings. It is necessary to define aggression because like other terms (e.g., motivation, confidence) it can be used in everyday language to describe a wide variety of behaviours. To illustrate, one American football coach may describe a player as aggressive if he tries to dominate his opponents at the scrimmage line. In contrast, a different American football coach may describe a player as aggressive if he makes deliberate attempts to injure opponents. This ambiguity of language that is common in everyday conversation is not tolerated in research. A clear definition of the variables under investigation enables research papers to be compared and studies to be replicated.

Remaining with aggression, we shall explore how an operational definition may be useful to a researcher seeking to reduce the frequency of aggressive behaviours in a youth soccer player. The researcher may adopt Baron and Richardson's (1994, p. 7) definition of aggression as 'any form of behaviour directed toward the goal of harming or injuring another living being who is motivated to avoid such treatment'. This definition is helpful as aggression is defined as a behaviour and as such it is observable. Further, the criteria of what the behaviour consists of are clear and, in addition to the more common physical actions, aggression can also incorporate psychological harm such as 'trash talking' and 'sledging' an opponent or official. Based on this definition, the researcher will likely derive a list of aggressive behaviours that will then be used to indicate aggression (e.g., late tackle, elbow in face, pushing, swearing at opponent). This definition and the list of aggressive behaviours will provide a way of quantifying behaviours that will enable other researchers to replicate the study so that the findings may be compared validly.

One limitation of operational definitions is that they will seldom cover all behaviours (Morgan and Morgan 2009). For example, in the case of aggression, the researcher would not be able to consider occasions when the player swears loudly and lashes out at the goalposts as behaving aggressively (as the intended victim must be living, based on the definition). Yet most people would consider such unsporting actions to be examples of aggressive behaviour. In addition, in our operational definition of aggression, there must be *intent* on behalf of the player to harm the victim either psychologically or physically – and determining intent can clearly be a difficult task as identical behaviours may be triggered by different intentions (e.g., the soccer player may hurt an opponent in a challenge because she intended to or because she mistimed the challenge). Accordingly, in this example there may be some behaviour that the researcher will have difficulty in classifying even when an operational definition is used. If this is the case, then whenever possible corroborating information can be used to help to 'triangulate' the data collection (i.e., validating the data collection process using two or more sources).

A second limitation of operational definitions outlined by Morgan and Morgan (2009) is that that they may have implications beyond the study when findings are communicated to the general public. Although researchers adopt a clear definition of a term, and this may be more precise than the way a term is used commonly, it is also important that the operational definition used in research relates to common usage. Again aggression in sport provides an excellent illustration of this. For many researchers, aggression is a moral issue and some psychologists would agree with the sentiments expressed by Tenenbaum, Sacks, Miller, Golden and Doolin (2000, p. 318) who suggested that 'behaviors intended to harm another are unacceptable in any contact or non-contact sport'. Yet for many athletes, it may be more accurate to say that aggression is a *necessary requirement* for success in many sports and furthermore much of the pleasure from playing contact sports may be derived from the physical contact and executing physically aggressive plays successfully (Kerr 1997). In short, although the International Society of Sport Psychology (ISSP) published a position statement outlining several ways in which violence and aggression in sport can be reduced (Tenenbaum, Stewart, Singer and Duda 1997), some athletes may relate more to the position espoused by Kerr (1999, 2002, 2005) that aggression is intrinsic and a pleasurable aspect of sport with the rules of many sports (e.g., boxing, ice hockey, rugby) allowing athletes to engage in behaviours that cause physical harm, and behaviours that can cause psychological harm (e.g., trash talking) are rarely legislated against. It could even be argued that athletes best equipped to harm opponents, physically and psychologically, within the rules of the sport, increase their chances of success. Therefore, a definition of aggression that does not recognize this point may lack credibility with some athletes and the public at large.

To summarize our discussion so far, behaviours to be measured in single-case research designs should be clearly defined and have a 'real-world' applicability that facilitates communication of the findings to the general public. These guidelines apply equally to other measures as well such as performance outcomes or psychological constructs. A clear definition of behaviour is essential for observers to collect data. Where possible, maintaining a record of the behaviour to be observed (e.g., through audio-visual recording) also enables the accuracy of the data to be checked and the data to be re-examined in the light of new developments. If this is not possible then a second observer could be employed in recording the behaviour as it happens. This secondary observer need not necessarily observe all sessions but can observe 20–30 per cent of the sessions to confirm the validity and reliability of the data collected by the primary observer and support the integrity of the research process (Morgan and Morgan 2009).

Although observation is important, single-case researchers should be aware that observing participants will likely bring about a change in behaviour – a phenomenon known as the 'Hawthorne effect'. It is to this effect that we now turn.

Hawthorne effect

The Hawthorne effect is an observation from a series of studies at the Hawthorne works of the Western Electric Company in Chicago that people changed their behaviour simply as a result of being observed (Whitehead 1938). The series of studies began in November 1924 to test the influence of brighter lighting on productivity (in this case assembling telephone relay switches) but the researchers discovered that both increasing and decreasing the lighting increased productivity, as did many other alterations to working conditions such as changes in hours and rest breaks (Gale 2004). That is, the increase in productivity was unrelated to changes in the physical environment or working conditions but rather seemed to occur because the environment was changed and the workers were subsequently observed. For the five assembly workers, the experience of being assessed and becoming the centre of attention actually changed their behaviour.

The Hawthorne effect is a challenge for single-case researchers because it suggests that, although observational data are important, the act of observation itself may actually change the behaviour under scrutiny. For example, in the domain of physical activity, a reluctant exerciser may increase his effort during his twice-weekly exercise class if he is being observed and a basketball player who responds with hostility to being penalized by officials may become more placid on being observed. It is difficult to suggest how a researcher may counteract this effect but, first, being *aware* that behaviour can change in response to being observed and, second, *triangulating* observed behaviour with accounts of behaviour when the participant was not being formally observed may help to tackle this problem. Furthermore, as Gale (2004) notes, the Hawthorne studies were conducted in 1920s America, a time and place in which the culture and experiences of the working class were different from what we know today, and this may limit the generalizability of the results. It was unusual at that time to pay such attention to the workers, who bonded as a group and gained autonomy, rewards and respect during participation in the study. It would not be surprising if these should be the over-riding factors in increasing productivity and the applicability of these findings to modern culture subsequently overstated. For example, it would be difficult to conceive of a professional sportsperson's behaviour being affected by the knowledge that he or she is being observed by someone specifically interested in his or her behaviour. This would, after all, not be an unusual occurrence.

In summary, the Hawthorne effect is something that single-case researchers should be aware of, and triangulation of data collected from the initial contact with information collated before any formal observation beginning is useful. For example, in the case of athletes, audio-visual recordings of past performance may form a useful way of collating information before formal observation begins.

So far in this chapter, we have discussed some broad issues about collecting data in single-case research. The type of data collected will depend on the specific aims of the proposed research and it is to the importance of clearly defining research aims that we now turn.

Defining research aims

In any form of empirical research, identifying the variables of interest is a crucial first step. Put simply, it is vital to be clear on what variables to manipulate [the independent variable(s)] or the specific nature of the intervention to deliver. In single-case research, the focus is usually on the latter. Of particular importance in single-case research is consideration of the dependent variable(s). The dependent variable(s) is the one that the researcher is interested in determining changes in over the course of the research. It is important to clearly define the dependent variable(s) and to determine what change in the dependent variable(s) is expected and desired. We shall now take each of these points in turn.

Defining the dependent variable

The variable of interest in single-case research might be a behaviour, an outcome, a psychological construct or a physiological change. The assessment and subsequent change of a desirable or undesirable behaviour is perhaps the most common approach in single-case research. To illustrate, Jones (1993) worked with an elite racket sport player and one aim of the intervention was to reduce the frequency of verbal outbursts towards the officials. This behaviour was undesirable because it distracted the player and Jones addressed this using a cognitive restructuring technique in which the participant was asked how many times in her career she had argued with officials (several hundred) and how many times this had resulted in a decision being changed (three or four). Based on this cognitive restructuring task the participant realized the futility of arguing with officials and was keen to commence a relaxation training programme to help her cope during times of frustration and reduce the verbal outbursts.

In addition to behaviours, there are other variables that may interest researchers and practitioners in sport and exercise. For example, rather than assessing a specific behaviour, the focus may be on a particular outcome such as unforced errors in athletic performance. To illustrate, Uphill and Jones (2005) used an intervention comprising imagery and task-focused instructions combined with an existing pre-shot routine to reduce the occurrence of 'careless shots' in an amateur golfer. These were shots in which the golfer considered he had made a simple error because he was not sufficiently focused, having been distracted by a previous error. The focus of this intervention was on a particular outcome (poor shot) that would relate to specific behaviours (e.g., swinging the club in a rushed manner).

Psychological constructs rather than a specific behaviour or outcome may also be the variable of interest. A psychological construct (e.g., anxiety, confidence, motivation, attitudes) is not something that can be observed directly but rather is inferred from other measures. Psychological constructs can be inferred from scores on self-report inventories including psychometric tests (e.g., an exerciser may complete a questionnaire indicating her enjoyment of exercise), from behaviours (e.g., posture may indicate confidence levels) or from physiological data (e.g., levels of cortisol may indicate anxiety). An illustration of how a psychological construct can form one of the primary dependent variables of interest in a single-case research design was provided by Barker and Jones (2006), who used hypnosis to enhance the self-efficacy of a cricket bowler.

Physiological aspects can also be the focus of interest in single-case research. A physiological variable may be assessed because a psychological construct can be inferred from the data (e.g., a hormone such as cortisol can be assessed as an operational index of levels of anxiety) or the physiological variable is the main aim of the research (e.g., reduction in cholesterol as a result of an exercise intervention). To illustrate how physiological data may be used in a single-case research design, Prapavessis, Grove, McNair and Cable (1992) reported how a twenty-year-old small-bore rifle shooter experienced debilitating levels of anxiety during competition. Following an intervention comprising relaxation strategies, thought stopping and biofeedback the levels of urinary adrenaline and noradrenaline (physiological markers indicative of anxiety) were lower in the shooter.

These examples of single-case research illustrate how different dependent variables (behaviours, outcomes, psychological constructs, physiological measures) can be part of the research design. Although a focus on one outcome measure is feasible, it is often pertinent to triangulate measures and this is frequently done. Triangulating data from different dependent variables in an intervention is important because it not only validates change but also helps to advance theoretical understanding by illustrating how certain variables may relate to each other. For example, Prapavessis et al. (1992) collected self-report measures of anxiety, performance measures and gun vibration in addition to the physiological measures, all of which indicated that a reduction in anxiety and a favourable influence on performance had occurred in the intervention with the rifle shooter. In a recent case study (as mentioned in Chapter 1), Barker and Jones (2008) explored the influence of a hypnosis intervention on self-efficacy, mood state and performance in a professional soccer player. In this instance, they were engaged in an intervention to enhance self-efficacy and positive mood because these constructs are associated with enhanced sport performance. If all three measures change in line with that expected following the intervention then there is greater certainty that the intervention has had the desired effect and the data provide further support for the association between self-efficacy, positive mood and performance.

In short, during single-case research it is desirable to collect as much data as possible to help understand the problem, validate the outcome and make a contribution to the research literature. Nevertheless, although collecting a range of data is important, not all data are equal. In the next section we consider the type of data that the single-case researcher is best focusing on and the type of data that best validate interventions and make a contribution to the literature.

What change is important? Establishing meaningful or statistical significance

As we shall explain later, data from single-case research can be analysed using visual analysis or statistical analysis (see Chapter 9). Traditional group-based research typically relies on statistical analysis of differences between average scores. In applied contexts, however, significant differences may not be appropriate or meaningful. So, in determining the change desired, the researcher should consider not only whether a difference is observed but also whether or not that change is *meaningful*. Considering the meaningfulness of results is familiar to researchers who are aware of the concept of effect size (see Cohen 1988). However, in the context of single-case research, detecting a meaningful change is not a *statistical* procedure. Instead, it is based on observing a change that has a tangible outcome. To illustrate, the guidelines from the American College of Sports Medicine and the American Heart Association (Haskell et al. 2007) state that adults should take part in five thirty-minute sessions of moderately intense physical activity per week. An exercise practitioner seeking to increase the physical activity levels of a sedentary client may consider any increase in physical activity to a level below these minimum levels to be clinically meaningless. If, for example, the participant has increased physical activity levels to three sessions of twenty-five minutes of physical activity a week this may represent a statistically significant increase in physical activity but still be one that falls below the minimum guidelines for health benefits. So, in that context, the change is not meaningful. Likewise, a tennis coach may seek to improve the first serve percentage of a junior international tennis player from a current level of 40 per cent. The tennis coach notices that similar players in the age group have a first serve percentage of around 65 per cent and introduces some modifications to the player's technique. The modifications do improve the first serve percentage but only to 50 per cent and so, although this change may be statistically significant, the resulting performance improvement is still well below what would be expected for a player in that age range. Of course, detecting a significant change and a meaningful change are not mutually exclusive. We do not suggest that researchers disregard statistical significance but where appropriate that consideration is always given to whether the changes refer to meaningful tangible outcomes.

Determining what is a meaningful change in behaviour or performance outcome is possible with any measure but there are particular challenges with self-report inventories. First, a participant's responses may be influenced by social desirability (a bias that occurs when people who are answering questions try to make themselves 'look good' instead of responding truthfully; Crowne and Marlowe 1960) and/or the demands of the experiment (from which the participant is able to guess what change is expected and responds accordingly, usually to 'help' the experimenter achieve the desired results; Orne 1962). That is, there is the possibility that the participant may complete an inventory in the way that they think is 'expected' or in the way 'that the researcher would like to see'. These outcomes may be particularly likely if the participant has built up a good relationship with the researcher and quite naturally would like to provide the 'right outcome'.

If inventories are completed honestly, then relating the scores to meaningful outcomes is still a challenge. It may be possible with inventories that have clearly defined norms and if there is a clear relationship between score and possible outcome. For example, a clinical psychologist may be working with an athlete who has suffered a career-threatening Achilles tendon injury. In this case, the athlete may exhibit symptoms of clinical depression and this is supported by a high score on the Beck Depression Inventory-II (BDI-II; Beck, Steer and Brown 1996), which indicates severe depression. The psychologist works with the participant and the score is reduced on the BDI-II as the participant progresses through the rehabilitation process, which indicates minimal depression. This may be accepted as a meaningful change in the participant's psychological state.

The difficulty with interpreting data collected from self-report measures is determining whether a meaningful change to a psychological state or behaviour also results in, and is concomitant to, the change observed on the inventory (Andersen, McCullagh and Wilson 2007). Even determining what the scores on inventories, such as the BDI-II, that are related to supposedly meaningful outcomes (such as less depressive behaviours and experiences) really mean for behaviours has been questioned (Andersen et al. 2007). For inventories with less clearly defined outcomes the problem is exacerbated. For example, what does a decrease of 10 points on the cognitive anxiety subscale of the CSAI-2 really equate to in terms of the participant's experience of anxiety? If an individual's score on the cognitive anxiety subscale is halved does that mean that they are half as worried as before? If cognitive anxiety impairs performance does a 10 per cent decrease in the cognitive anxiety subscale of the CSAI-2 equate to a 10 per cent increase in performance? The issue of the meaningfulness of scores on measures has been termed arbitrary metrics and a metric (i.e., the measure employed) is defined as arbitrary if 'it is not known where a given score locates an individual on the underlying psychological dimension or how a one-unit change on the observed score reflects the magnitude of change on the underlying dimension' (Blanton and Jaccard 2006, p. 28).

Moreover, if we accept Andersen et al.'s (2007, p. 665) premise that 'the central outcomes of health, sport, and exercise interventions should still primarily be behaviours in the real world' then it poses a challenge to single-case researchers. Specifically, if only self-report measures are taken how should these relate to clearly observable tangible changes that relate to meaningful effects, specifically observable behaviours. If the measures taken do not incorporate observable behaviours, nor do they include measures that can be clearly equated with observable behaviours, then the research lacks validity. Of course, as Andersen et al. (2007) warned, we must be careful when discussing the meaningfulness of variables. To illustrate, in sport, winning and losing is not always the same as success or failure (in a scientific sense) because these outcomes can be influenced by factors outside of the participant's control and crucially may not be an accurate reflection of the behaviours or constructs in which the researcher is interested.

To summarize, it is necessary to clearly define the variables to assess and determine what is considered a meaningful change. Of particular importance in determining a meaningful change is relating change to observable behaviour in sport and exercise settings, or that the change itself should be an observable behaviour (Andersen et al. 2007). The focus of the chapter now moves to consider how change is determined. Particular focus must be devoted to baseline data that enable change to be determined.

The baseline

In order to determine change (statistical, meaningful or both) it is necessary to collect baseline data. Baseline data provide the standard by which any subsequent change can be compared and in the case of an intervention its efficacy can be determined. In a baseline, the frequency and/or intensity of the variable(s) of interest are recorded. If an intervention is to be deployed, then baseline collection of data will also inform the intervention to be delivered. Two key considerations in designing and evaluating a baseline are its stability and its length (Barlow et al. 2009).

Baseline stability

The stability of the baseline is crucial because an unstable and highly variable baseline does not enable the researcher to draw a meaningful comparison with any subsequent data. If the data are stable, as indicated in Figure 3.1, then it makes determining a meaningful change easier. However, the data may be highly variable (see Figure 3.2) or there may be a trend in the data in a particular direction (see Figures 3.3 and 3.4).

As Barlow et al. (2009) noted, the task of classifying the level of stability required is not simple – and there are no agreed guidelines that can be applied across all situations. For a start, some types of behaviour or outcomes are likely to vary substantially by virtue of their transient nature. To illustrate, as we have shown in Figure 3.2, the number of runs scored by a cricket batsman can vary substantially given the fact that dismissal can be influenced by a number of factors – including pitch conditions, poor decision making by the officials, good performance by the bowler and simply luck! In contrast the times run by a 100-metre sprinter, although variable, are likely to be a more consistent reflection of performance level (see Figure 3.1), but even these may vary as the sprinter progresses through her normal training cycle. Also, it is possible that variability in the behaviour observed may result from environmental changes

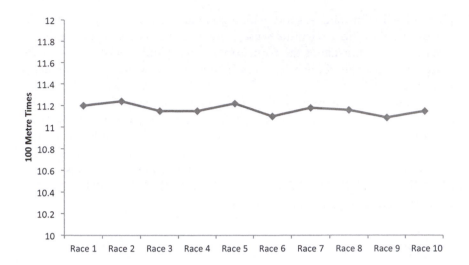

FIGURE 3.1 A stable baseline – hypothetical race time data from a female 100-metre runner.

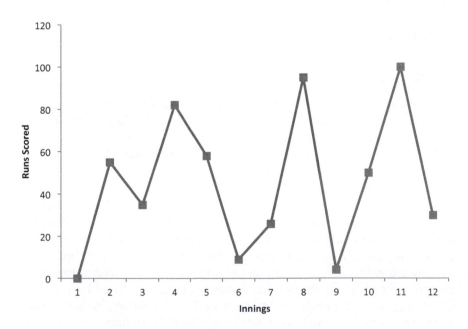

FIGURE 3.2 A variable baseline – hypothetical data on the runs scored by a county cricket batsman.

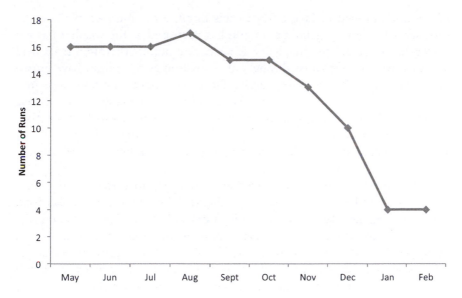

FIGURE 3.3 A decreasing baseline – hypothetical data on the number of times per month a recreational exerciser went jogging.

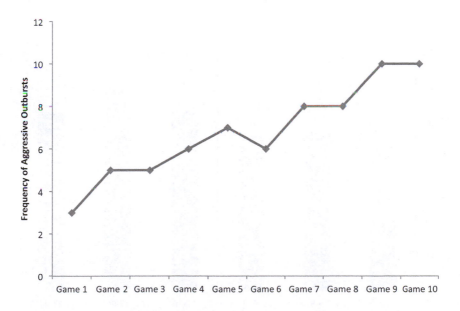

FIGURE 3.4 An increasing baseline – hypothetical data on the number of aggressive outbursts towards officials per game for a male field hockey player.

as we have outlined in Figure 3.3. In this instance the number of times the participant has gone jogging per month has decreased as the weather has got colder. In Figure 3.4 the frequency of aggressive outbursts from a male field hockey player has increased throughout the season as the games have grown more important. Clearly, understanding the data collected, and how these may vary, is important. In addition to the examples of variability and trends we have outlined in Figures 3.1–3.4, there are many other types of variability that are combinations of the patterns we have presented. For example, it is possible for a baseline to be first stable, then variable and vice versa. Likewise, data may first increase then decrease.

If the data are inherently variable then it may help to average them and to present them in blocks. For example, in Figure 3.5 we revisit the cricket batsman's performance data presented in Figure 3.2. This graph reports both the baseline data and also data collected after an intervention that was administered by the cricket batsman's coach and involved him changing his stance at the crease slightly as he waited for the ball. In this graph we have blocked the data into the average number of runs scored per four innings to help eliminate the variability in the data and facilitate comparison with the post-intervention data.

Had the data not been blocked they would have appeared as in Figure 3.6. Determining change from the highly variable data set outlined in this figure is clearly a challenge and explains why the data were averaged in Figure 3.5 – because it makes the interpretation of the data easier and removes some of the

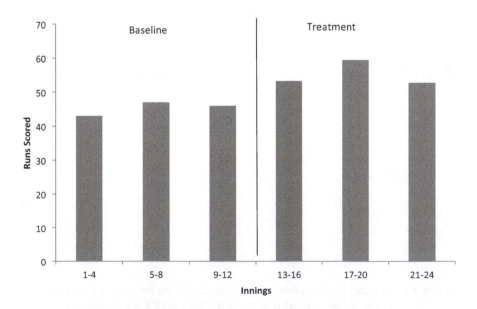

FIGURE 3.5 Averaged data – hypothetical data on the runs scored by a county cricket batsman before and after an intervention to alter his stance.

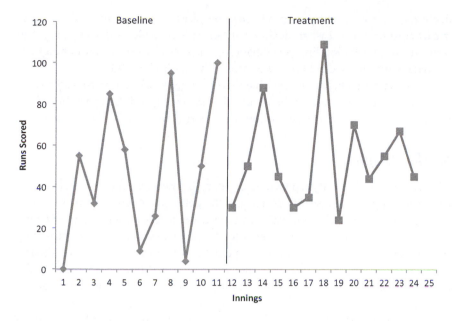

FIGURE 3.6 Variable data – hypothetical data on the runs scored by a county cricket batsman before and after an intervention to alter his stance.

variability inherent in run scoring (even the best cricket batsman will occasionally score few runs).

Not all single-case researchers may agree with our averaging strategy, however. For example, Kazdin (1982) suggested caution in treating the data this way. First, the variability of the data may actually indicate important information. For example, in Figure 3.6 it is possible to observe that not only does the cricket batsman score more runs but also he becomes more consistent and there is less variability in his performance after the intervention. Also averaging the data reduces the number of data points, which may be problematic if the averaged data do not produce a stable baseline.

Variability, or a trend, in the baseline can be problematic as it makes determining a meaningful change after the intervention difficult. For example, the guidelines for visual analysis outlined in Chapter 9 suggest that overlap between data points (which is more likely with variable data) makes drawing conclusions through visual analysis difficult. Indeed, when variability exceeds 50 per cent the use of statistics would be considered appropriate (Barlow et al. 2009). However, as outlined in Chapter 9, variability or a trend in the data does not make determining meaningful changes impossible (of course, it depends to a degree on the extremity of any variability or trend). Analysis of the data can consider the trend line and reversing an increase in an undesirable outcome could of course be seen as a success. For example, an individual with a steadily declining exercise participation rate may be pleased (at least for a short time) if participation rates cease to decline further. It is possible to detect changes in trend using a celeration line (see Chapters 5 and 9) and a minimum of eight to ten data points are needed for this approach (Ottenbacher 1986).

Where data are likely to be variable then a longer baseline is necessary to give an accurate representation of the issue to be addressed, and the variability of the baseline cannot be considered without considering the length of the baseline.

Baseline length

The issue of baseline length provides another illustration of the tension between the strongest possible research design and the demands of working in an applied setting where practical circumstances may upset a researcher's plans. Having approached someone (the researcher) for help, a participant may be unwilling to undergo a lengthy period of assessment before an intervention takes place. Clearly, practitioners should only intervene with a proper evaluation of the problem (see Heyman 1987), but a lengthy baseline is not always necessary to provide an appropriate evaluation of a problem. The purpose of the baseline is to provide the standard by which any subsequent change can be compared and, in the case of an intervention, its efficacy can be determined. So a baseline should first provide an *accurate* indication of frequency and/or intensity of the variable(s) of interest and be sufficiently stable to enable a meaningful comparison. When collecting data, a whole host of variables may influence the frequency or intensity of a particular variable (e.g., standard of opponent, teammates, weather). The greater the number of potential influences on the variable and the greater the natural variation in the variable of interest the longer the baseline should be to provide an indication of stability. We recognize that failing to provide definitive guidelines as to the stability or length of a baseline might seem unhelpful. However, rather than following specific criteria the important factor is that a baseline should provide an accurate indication of frequency and/ or intensity of the variable(s) of interest and be sufficiently stable to enable a meaningful comparison.

To conclude, baseline data provide the standard by which change, or the efficacy of an intervention, can be determined. The baseline should provide a stable, accurate indication of frequency and/or intensity of the variable(s) of interest, and because variables differ in their stability then baseline length will not be consistent across all single-case research. We now turn to consider issues involved in determining change from the baseline.

Issues in determining change

Determining a behavioural change to be both meaningful and interpretable requires the researcher to have considered in detail the implementation of the intervention or the way in which the independent variable was manipulated.

More precisely, the researcher should be able to understand the natural variation in the data, present the data appropriately and, on the basis of the presentation, interpret the changes in the data after baseline.

Change one variable at a time

Barlow et al. (2009) suggested that a cardinal rule of single-case research is to change *only one variable* when moving from one phase to another. To explain, if after a baseline phase (A) in which attendance at the gym was monitored, a fitness instructor introduces personal targets for a reluctant gym user along with greater personal attention when using the equipment and then monitors gym attendance during the intervention phase (B) it is not possible to determine what brought about any observed change in behaviour. There is nothing wrong with using both these techniques as an intervention simultaneously in an applied setting but there are obvious difficulties in using different techniques simultaneously as an intervention in a research paper. We have been guilty of this in our past research. For example, we used hypnosis and self-modelling to enhance the self-efficacy and performance of a cricket bowler (Barker and Jones 2006). As an applied intervention, this was perfectly acceptable and both self-efficacy and performance increased in the cricketer. However, for researchers interested in causal relationships, our study had limitations. Specifically, it was not possible to determine from the intervention whether the hypnosis or the self-modelling made the greater contribution. Similar examples abound in the sport and exercise literature, in particular in sport psychology in which there is a tendency for researchers to use multi-modal interventions in working with clients (e.g., Freeman, Rees and Hardy 2009; Prapavessis et al. 1992; Thelwell and Greenlees 2003). Multi-modal interventions may reflect how applied work is conducted with a client, and *are* therefore worthy of research, but the data collected can only be taken to reflect the particular combination of techniques used if a simple A–B design is used. It will not provide as much information as a study in which the introduction of each variable is monitored on an individual basis, in, for example, an A–B–A–C–A–B–C design. To illustrate, consider the cricket bowler who was the focus of the intervention by Barker and Jones (2006). In this instance, the research could have been structured such that A would be the baseline, B is hypnosis and C is self-modelling. After the baseline phase hypnosis is introduced then removed, self-modelling is introduced then removed and finally both interventions are re-introduced. This is clearly a stronger research design but one that is difficult to achieve in an applied setting.

Natural variation

There will likely be a natural variation in the data that the researchers should be aware of when interpreting change. One particular type of variation pertinent to single-case research is regression, which is the tendency for a behaviour to revert to normal. Perhaps the best known example of regression is provided by Kahneman and Tversky (1973) who presented a scenario, based on personal experience, of instructors in a flight training school who concluded that positive reinforcement after successful execution of a complex flight manoeuvre led to worse performance on the next performance of the manoeuvre. The flight instructors made this conclusion having observed that after executing a complex move well (and quite naturally being praised for it) performance on a subsequent attempt of the manoeuvre was worse. However, as Kahneman and Tversky explained, this type of regression in performance (after a successful execution of a complex manoeuvre) was inevitable because progress on learning a complex task is rarely smooth and pilots who did exceptionally well in one trial were *likely* to deteriorate on the next attempt regardless of the feedback from the instructors. In short, performance was likely to regress after an excellent performance in someone still learning a skill regardless of the comments offered by the instructors.

Understanding regression effects is important in single-case research because, as Kazdin (1982) noted, a researcher may obtain an extreme data point during the baseline phase that is in the opposite direction to that anticipated after the intervention. If this extreme data point is at the end of the baseline phase, then when the data regress to typical values after the intervention then it may artificially inflate the effect of the intervention and suggest an improvement that is a result of regression and not the intervention. If an extreme score occurs, it may be best not to change phases at that point.

Assessing long-term change

A crucial challenge in intervention research is the issue of determining the degree to which any change observed is genuine. There is a possibility that any differences may be a result of observation, as the Hawthorne researchers discovered, social desirability (Crowne and Marlowe 1960) or experimental demands (Orne 1962). An improvement could also be a placebo effect, whereby the intervention administered has the desired effect not because it has any inherent value in addressing the specific issue but because the participant believes it will work. One way in which the researcher can have greater confidence in the efficacy of any intervention is to assess its effect over the longer term.

We do not suggest that the Hawthorne effect, social desirability, experimental demands or the placebo effect cannot influence behaviour in the long term. Instead, we consider it less likely that they will do so. It is *more likely* that, if the intervention has had a genuine effect, long-term maintenance effects will be observed because the issue of concern has been addressed. To explain, if the participant has changed behaviour, not because the intervention worked, but because of a belief that the intervention was useful, then the underlying issues are likely to emerge at a later time point. In short, the participant has not fundamentally changed. To illustrate how follow-up long-term data can be collected in single-case research, Barker and Jones (2006) monitored the effects of a hypnosis and self-modelling intervention to enhance the self-efficacy and performance of a cricket bowler over the second half of the cricket season and also collected data from the first half of the subsequent season to check that the gains observed were maintained into the subsequent season. Regardless of how the data are collected, and for how long, the interpretation of the data will be influenced by the presentation. Let us now consider the importance of graphical representation.

The importance of graphical representation

Visual inspection of graphical data is the most widely used and easily understood method of data analysis for single-case research (Ottenbacher 1986; see also Chapter 9). In this section, we outline some key issues to consider in the presentation and interpretation of figures in single-case research.

Figures 3.1–3.4 are examples of simple line graphs, which are the simplest and most frequent method of data analysis. The horizontal x-axis is typically divided according to units of observation (e.g., trials, matches, games) or time (e.g., months). The vertical y-axis refers to the unit of measurement of the dependent variable. Although a line graph is often used it is possible to present the data in a bar graph (e.g., Figures 3.5 and 3.7). A bar graph can show the magnitude of change, particularly if it represents the mean of each phase as Figure 3.7 does.

However, as already noted, plotting data in this manner does not indicate the trend of the data, nor the variability, which is important information necessary to understand change. To convey the information accurately, the graphs must be properly constructed and three key points, outlined by Ottenbacher (1986), include (1) different phases should be clearly delineated (e.g., using a bold vertical or dashed vertical line); (2) a graph can contain more then one data path (i.e., set of data), but this can be confusing so no more than three data paths should be included on any one graph and the line should be clearly delineated using geometric forms; and (3) the graph should be labelled clearly and logically and the scaling system should be simple and easy to read.

Determining a meaningful and interpretable change requires the researcher to understand the implementation of the intervention or the manipulation of an independent variable and, further, to be aware that natural variation in the data may artificially inflate the effect of the intervention and suggest an improvement that is a result of regression and not the intervention. The strengths of the conclusions drawn from the research can be enhanced with the use of long-term follow-up data, and where possible this should be done. Finally, it is important for researchers to present the data appropriately in a manner that facilitates interpretation of changes in the data after baseline.

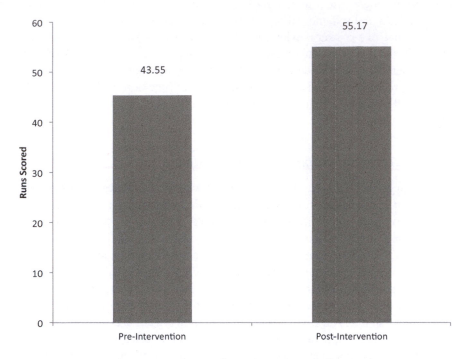

FIGURE 3.7 Pre- and post-intervention data – hypothetical data on the average runs scored by a county cricket batsman before and after an intervention to alter his stance.

Summary

In this chapter we have highlighted some of the ways in which the quality of single-case research can be compromised and conversely how it can be enhanced. The issues covered are not only those we consider valuable for those involved in single-case research but also those that are applicable for the field as a whole in critically evaluating the research conducted.

Key points

• Determine before starting the intervention what changes are the focus of the research, and the meaningfulness of the changes.
• Be confident that the baseline provides an accurate and as far as possible stable representation of the variables.
• Behaviours to be observed should be clearly defined.
• Be aware of how the Hawthorne effect, social desirability, experimental demands and the placebo effect may influence results and where possible limit the influence by collecting long-term follow-up data.

- Be aware of natural variation in the data and how that can influence the perception of a change.
- Present data in a clear graphical format.

Guided study

Based on your reading of Chapter 3 please take some time to respond to the following review questions:

- What are the key issues surrounding data collection in single-case research?
- Explain the Hawthorne effect and comment on how this potential issue can be minimized.
- Discuss which is more important in applied single-case research: meaningful or statistical significance.
- Explain the major facets of collecting baseline data.
- Explain how change can be determined in single-case research.

4

ASSESSING BEHAVIOUR IN SPORT AND EXERCISE

In this chapter, we will:

- explain the rationale for assessing behaviour in sport and exercise;
- outline some key methods by which we can assess behaviour;
- illustrate these behaviour assessment methods in sport and exercise contexts.

Introduction

Most practitioners in sport and exercise focus on producing predictable and replicable improvements in behaviour. The behaviour(s), however, is not chosen randomly. Instead, practitioners tend to choose socially significant behaviour with short- and long-term benefits for the sport performer and those who interact with that sport performer (Cooper, Heron and Heward 2007). For example, working together, a practitioner and client might identify lateness for squad training as the target behaviour that should be addressed to benefit the sport performer and the squad. Many practitioners in sport and exercise aspire to change a client's behaviour either directly or indirectly. But to change a client's behaviour, the practitioner must first identify the specific behaviour targeted for change; next, specify the parameters of that behaviour; and, finally, measure that behaviour. Without guiding principles to assess behaviour, it becomes difficult to monitor and evaluate professional practice and justify that the treatment explained the behaviour change rather than any other factor. The most valid measure to assess change in a client's behaviour is to observe the client's behaviour. If, for example, you want to understand how many times a rugby player verbally criticizes other rugby players in her team, you can observe that rugby player's verbal criticisms at practice and competition. Practitioners manage behavioural observation by sampling the client's behaviour over time or situation and they use various instruments to record behaviour. This chapter builds on the issues surrounding behavioural assessment raised in Chapter 3 and will examine why practitioners need to assess behaviour in sport and exercise and how behaviours are selected, defined and measured.

Selecting and defining behaviours to assess

Behaviour represents what people do (e.g., time spent training) rather than the characteristics that people may have (e.g., confidence; Bloom, Fischer and Orme 2009). It includes a complex variety of thoughts, feelings and actions (Friman 2009). In general, human behavioural activities may be either overt or covert. Overt events are things that can be observed by others such as the number of laps a swimmer completes at the pool or the number of times a week a golfer practises putting. Covert events, however, occur within the individual and so cannot be observed directly by others. Typical of such activities are the amount of times a gymnast feels anxious before a competition or the number of self-deprecating thoughts a badminton player has during a badminton game. The challenge for the practitioner, therefore, is to recognize that behaviour must be observable and measurable by someone, either the client or an external observer (Bloom et al. 2009).

Behavioural assessment fulfils a vital role in sport and exercise research because it allows the researcher to identify, change and monitor a behaviour or set of behaviours over time. A sport psychologist might value identifying those behaviours that prevent a snooker player from excelling in a competitive match. Those behaviours might include irregular pre-pot routines and self-deprecating post-pot evaluations. Once these behaviours are identified as typically occurring in a competitive match, the sport psychologist can help the snooker player to modify those behaviours and help him to engage in a stable routine regardless of shot demands and establish at least one positive aspect of his preparation for the pot, regardless of the outcome. The sport psychologist can monitor the behaviour of the snooker player, especially his pre-pot routine and post-pot evaluations, to determine whether a change has occurred in his behaviour.

Applied behaviour analysis focuses on significant social or applied behaviours (Baer, Wolf and Risley 1968; Kazdin 1982; Kratochwill 2007). These behaviours are almost endless in sport and exercise contexts and include such diverse activities as tardiness for practice sessions, skill learning and aggression. We can consider many applied or socially significant behaviours that are worth assessing, such as those that are important to a client (e.g., performing successfully in competition) or behaviours (e.g., aggression, bulimia) that might be dangerous to the client or to others. But it is not always obvious which behaviour to address or which behaviour offers the greatest reward for the client and the community (Kazdin 1982). Wolf (1978) proposed that clients and those in contact with the client value the methods, goals and outcomes of an intervention. In other words, we assess a study's social validity by the appropriateness of the procedures, the social significance of the target behaviour and the social importance of the results (Cooper et al. 2007). Those directly (e.g., client) and indirectly (e.g., family members, coach, teammates) involved in the intervention can rate these three criteria of a behaviour change programme. Even when a client's verbal statements suggest a treatment was effective, we cannot assume that this was the case because 'a subject's verbal description of his own nonverbal behaviour usually would not be accepted as a measure of his actual behaviour' (Baer et al. 1968, p. 93). In the next section we shall explain social comparison and subjective evaluation. Together these assessments inform us about the consumer satisfaction of a behaviour change programme (Hawkins 1979).

Social comparison

Social comparison allows practitioners to validate the social significance of behaviour changes. They can use several methods to achieve this aim (Cooper et al. 2007). First, they can compare a client's performance with the performance of a normative sample. In this method, a peer group of the client is identified (e.g., an exercise class, a basketball team). This peer group would be similar to the client because they perform similar actions (e.g., exercise, play basketball) with similar demographics but differ in the target behaviour being assessed. Practitioners can gather normative data about the particular behaviour before the intervention and use the behaviour of the client's peer group as a normative sample. Second, they can ask consumers to rate the social validity of participants' performance, which is also referred to as subjective evaluation. In this process the opinions of others are sought because of their expertise or familiarity with the client. These people can judge or evaluate the behaviours in need of treatment (Kazdin 1982). Sometimes an intervention is sought because consensus develops among a coaching team that a particular behaviour is problematic. For instance, Collins, Morriss and Trower (1999) described how the coaching team of an elite javelin thrower invited sport science support to help the javelin thrower rediscover particular positions at crucial positions of the throw. In this intervention, the athlete, coach and biomechanist collaborated with the sport psychologist to regain a lost move.

Martin and Hrycaiko (1983) suggested that coaches should regularly question athletes, parents and others in the sport environment to evaluate how they feel about dimensions of the coaching programme. When athletes get an opportunity to express how they feel about particular aspects of a coaching programme, it is possible to generate better outcomes for everyone. They also suggested that those involved in the intervention should have a chance to express their satisfaction with the results obtained. Practitioners can use standardized tests to assess the social validity of behaviour change programme outcomes. Finally, assessing the client's behaviour in the natural environment probably provides the most socially valid assessment of a client's newly learned behaviour. In sport, we might observe the client in competition, a real-world test of social validity.

For any intervention in sport and exercise, the goal is to return the person or people to a particular level of functioning (Kazdin 1982). The two elements constituting social validation, social comparison and subjective evaluation, have been used occasionally in sport and exercise settings. Although they provide empirically based procedures for systematically selecting target behaviours for assessment and intervention, Kazdin (1977) also identified some problems in this field. To begin with, even if a client differs from her peer group on a particular behaviour, it does not mean that the behaviour is important or that resolving the differences in performance will solve the major problems for the client. Also, even when consensus among peers about a particular behaviour exists, this behaviour might not be the most important focus of treatment. In sport and exercise contexts, this might represent the team you compete alongside. At least three questions should be posed about interventions in sport and exercise (Martin et al. 2004, p. 275): (1) What do participants (and perhaps significant others) think about the goals of the intervention? (2) What do they think about the procedures that were applied? (3) What do they think about the results produced by those procedures? Most studies in sport and exercise contexts include these questions, or a variation of these questions, and pose them to the client after the intervention. For instance, Mellalieu, Hanton and Thomas (2009) examined the effects of a motivational general-arousal imagery intervention upon pre-performance symptoms in male rugby union players. These authors asked participants to respond anonymously to a post-intervention social validation questionnaire to establish the practical effectiveness of the intervention. The participants responded on a 1 (not at all) to 7 (extremely) Likert scale to four questions: (1) How important to you is improvement on the performance component that you have selected? (2) Do you consider any of the performance changes that have occurred to be significant? (3) How satisfied are you with the intervention? and (4) Has the procedure proved useful to you? These authors also used an open-ended question for the participants to explain their reasons for the success or failure of the intervention. Wolko, Hrycaiko and Martin (1993) investigated the effects of adding a private and public self-management package to standard coaching among five young female gymnasts. Both self-management packages were effective in improving the practice performance of gymnasts with private self-regulation being the most effective technique. They extended the subjective evaluation of the results by surveying gymnastic coaches. These coaches perceived the gymnasts' skill development as significantly improved with the private self-regulation package.

In summary, behavioural assessment in sport and exercise offers many benefits to sport performers, exercisers and coaches, among others (Tkachuk, Leslie-Toogood and Martin 2003). First, aspects of the environment that influence problem behaviour can be identified and changed during a treatment programme. Second, rather than perceiving possible behaviour change because of an intervention, accurate records of behaviour demonstrate the effectiveness of a treatment programme. On their own, recording and charting behaviour might produce improvements (e.g., McKenzie and Rushall 1974). Charted improvements in a behaviour signal a powerful incentive to continue with the treatment and recognize the value of the treatment. Finally, the evidence gained from behavioural assessment can be used to meet standards of professional accountability (Smith 1988). A thorough behavioural assessment establishes a roadmap from which the variables controlling the behaviour can be identified and understood, allowing subsequent interventions to focus on targets that generate success (Cooper et al. 2007).

Measuring behaviour

A central tenet of single-case designs is the importance of assessing accurately the occurrence of the target behaviour or the specific activity to be changed (Tkachuk et al. 2003). As discussed in Chapter 3 the investigator must carefully define the target variable or behaviour to observe, especially if more than one person is asked to report on the target variable or behaviour. Only when the target behaviour is explicitly defined can those involved in the treatment observe and measure that behaviour to implement treatment. This assessment strategy is necessary for at least two reasons. First, so that the performance of the target behaviour can be identified before the intervention begins. In single-case designs, this is referred to as a baseline. Second, so that, after the intervention begins, those assessing the behaviour can record the change. In this way, the altered behaviour can be compared with the baseline behaviour.

Changing behaviour is an arduous task. Martin and Hrycaiko (1983) explained that effective behavioural coaching requires (1) precise definition of the behaviours that are critical to success for athletes; (2) accurate and frequent recording of aspects of those behaviours before, during and after behavioural interventions; and (3) consistent and individualized application of specific behaviour modification procedures. Hawkins (1979) suggested that behavioural assessment can be considered to form a funnel with a broad scope followed by a narrow and constant focus. The behavioural assessment comprised five phases: (1) screening and general disposition, (2) defining and generally quantifying the problem or achievement, (3) pinpointing and designing of intervention, (4) monitoring progress and (5) follow up. Although presented in a chronological order, their functions are not limited in time because the functions of each phase often overlap.

Three criteria must be met to satisfy the target response: objectivity, clarity and completeness (Hawkins and Dobes 1977; Kazdin 1982). Objectivity is achieved when the definition of the target behaviour refers to observable characteristics of behaviour or environmental events. Clarity is achieved when the definition is unambiguous for observers to understand. Completeness is achieved when the definition has enough information to determine what behaviour should be included and excluded. If the boundaries are loose, observers will have to infer whether a response occurred. For instance, if we are recording non-verbal coaching behaviour, specific definitions should allow each observer to accurately record the non-verbal coaching behaviour of the coach. Sage advice beckons us to observe the client informally. Descriptive notes of what behaviours occur and which events are associated with their occurrence may be useful in generating specific response definitions.

Many of the behaviours we observe in sport and exercise contexts are associated with other events and so do not occur in a vacuum. For instance, the verbal behaviour of a teammate might influence the verbal behaviour of the client. However, verbal behaviour is but one influence; gestures (e.g., pat on the back) and facial expressions (e.g., smiles, frowns) may also influence performance and these stimuli may precede or follow the target behaviour (Kazdin 1982). This is most likely in a coaching environment. Most researchers' and practitioners' observations emerge from directly observing overt performances. But these are not the only strategies for collecting data about the target behaviour. Other strategies that we will discuss later include self-report and psychophysiological assessments that are specific to the target behaviour. Some sport psychologists, for example, use biofeedback to help performers understand what happens to their bodies when they become anxious (see Davis and Sime 2005). We will begin, however, by exploring overt behaviour.

Sport and exercise practitioners have four major methods to obtain assessment information. Two methods – interviews and checklists – are indirect because the data emerge from recollections or subjective ratings of events. Two methods – tests and direct observation – are direct because they inform us about a person's behaviour as it occurs (Cooper et al. 2007). In professional practice, sport psychologists often interview clients at the beginning of a professional relationship to understand how they can assist the client. These interviews may occur face to face or over the telephone and have specific functions to determine whether further consultation is possible (Katz and Hemmings 2009). In a behavioural interview, the behaviour analyst asks *what* and *how* questions to understand the environmental conditions that exist before, during and after a behavioural episode. *Why* questions are avoided because such questions presume that the client knows the answer to the question, causing frustration because they probably do not know the answer (Kadushin 1972). Behaviour checklists and rating scales are often combined with interviews to identify the target behaviour. Such measures can help to identify behaviours that require a direct assessment.

Direct observation

When practitioners measure overt behaviour they usually measure how often a discrete response occurs (i.e., frequency) or the amount of time for which the response occurs (i.e., rate). With a frequency measure, the practitioner counts the number of times the behaviour occurs in a certain amount of time. This task is relatively easy if you are counting the number of strokes a swimmer takes to complete one length of the swimming pool. When the action is discrete, there is a clear beginning and end to that behaviour and it should occur in a similar amount of time, each time. In this way, each unit is comparable. But, for example, if a coach were engaging in ongoing behaviours, such as talking to his players, counting the number of times he speaks to his players would not accurately reflect that behaviour because he might speak with one player for ten seconds and another player for thirty seconds. By counting the instances only, you omit the vital information about duration.

If the times are not comparable, frequency measures deny us accurate information about behaviour. In this case we need to assess the rate of response by dividing the frequency of responses by the number of minutes observed. This practice supplies a frequency rate per minute. Kazdin (1982) demonstrated some useful features of the frequency measure for practitioners. First, it is a relatively simple method to apply in natural settings and we can operate counters when recording. Second, frequency measures reveal changes over time in a particular behaviour. The goal of many programmes is to increase or decrease the number of times a particular behaviour occurs and frequency measures supply that direct measure. We might be interested in how often one team successfully tackles members of another team in rugby. Such frequency scores can deliver this information. If we seek to measure two or more behaviours, we can also do that by discrete categorization. In other words, we can measure different behaviours that have occurred or not when they have a clear beginning and end and are of a similar duration. In a sport setting, a practitioner might apply discrete categorization to measure the number of successful passes and tackles made by a defender. For each game, the behaviours on the checklist could be categorized as performed or not performed and the total number of behaviours performed correctly constitutes the measure of effective play. Because sports such as football, basketball or rugby are difficult to assess in performance terms, more sensitive measures are required beyond win–loss records and goals or points scored. Komaki and Barnett (1977) used a behavioural approach to coach a Pop Warner football team (youth American football) to reduce the emphasis on winning and address the lack of frequent and contingent reinforcement. The authors classified three frequently run offensive plays into a series of five behaviourally defined stages with checklists to observe players in practice and competition. This checklist allowed both the coach and the players to assess and offer frequent and contingent consequences for desired execution of skills. Each act performed correctly was scored. The reinforcement programme increased the number of steps completed correctly. Without the behavioural specification, it would be difficult to determine whether the desired skills were executed properly and, based on this execution, to provide positive reinforcement.

Galvan and Ward (1998) set up a single-subject multiple-baseline design across five players to assess the effectiveness of public posting in reducing inappropriate on-court behaviours in collegiate tennis players. The response class included four abuse categories: racquet (when a player threw or struck an object with the racquet), verbal (when a player screamed negative comments at spectators, teammates or umpires), ball (when the player threw or struck the ball other than to play tennis) and physical (when the player displayed self-injurious behaviour such as slapping or pulling hair). In this study, these behaviours were counted and aggregated for each set and averaged across the number of sets in a challenge match. This intervention, involving feedback on inappropriate behaviours, goal setting and public posting, immediately reduced the inappropriate on-court behaviours for all players.

Certain behaviours are required by all team members to perform correctly and produce the desired performance for the team. We might assess the team's tardiness. When we define the desired behaviour (see Chapter 3), we can assess how many of the team perform the desired behaviour. Similar to the treatment of frequency and categorization measures, the observer can classify whether the response occurred or not. In this setting, it is the *individuals* who are counted rather than the number of times the individual performs the response (Kazdin 1982). The problem with this type of measure is that is does not offer specific information about the performance of a particular individual. For example, Shearer, Mellalieu, Shearer and Roderique-Davies (2009) used a multiple-baseline across-groups design to examine the effects of an imagery intervention on perceptions of collective efficacy. Ten members of an international wheelchair basketball team were separated into three regional intervention groups. Each group completed a similar intervention comprising a four-week, video-aided, motivational general-mastery imagery programme. One group's collective efficacy increased, another group became more consistent and there were no changes in the final group.

Interval recording

Researchers and practitioners in sport and exercise use two time-based measurements: interval recording and response duration. Interval recording focuses on units of time rather than on units of discrete response. Behaviour is recorded during a short period (e.g., thirty minutes per training session) rather than for the total time that it is performed (Kazdin 1982), and this block of time can be divided into a series of short intervals. For example, an observer might record the client's behaviour in intervals of fifteen seconds. During these intervals, the target behaviour is scored as having occurred or not occurred. Kazdin (1982) suggested that, when a discrete behaviour such as striking an opponent occurs more than once in a single interval, that response is scored as having occurred; that is, when a response occurs again in the same interval, it is not counted separately.

In sport, for example, a sport psychologist might assess whether a player is paying attention and working diligently on a task in practice. The practitioner would use interval recording to record the player's behaviour at intervals of fifteen seconds over a fifteen-minute observational period. For example, an observer could record whether a golfer works in his driving range bay at intervals of fifteen seconds for fifteen minutes. If the golfer remains in the bay working on his ball-striking skills, many intervals will be scored for attentive behaviour. If, however, the golfer stops work and chats to others around him, then inattentive behaviour will be scored. Because each interval is scored for attentive or inattentive behaviour, strict guidelines must apply because the golfer taking a rest might be engaging in useful discussion with a colleague. Another challenge that the observer encounters is recording many behaviours in an interval because this takes time and attention, which is also required for observing the client. The observer needs more time to record behaviour, especially if the observer began recording behaviour before the end of the interval (Kazdin 1982). In this instance, an observer might use interval-scoring procedures that allow time to record after each interval of observation. In our example above, we might take ten seconds of observation and five seconds to record these observations after the interval. Short recording times are best because, when the observer is recording behaviour, no behaviour is being observed.

In summary, interval recording is valuable in sport and exercise contexts because it is flexible and most behaviour can be recorded (Kazdin 1982). The simplicity of classifying the target behaviour as occurring or not occurring during a short period reduces the burden on the observer. To aid analysis, we can yield percentages of behaviours occurring or not occurring. For example, if an attentive behaviour occurs twenty times in eighty intervals observed, the percentage of intervals of attentive behaviour is 25 per cent. This method is useful for coaches or psychologists to understand the occurrence or lack of occurrence of the target behaviour. If the behaviour is continuous, the observer can record the amount of time that the response is performed. This duration method is useful for programmes trying to increase or decrease the length of time of a particular response.

Self-report and self-monitoring

Although many studies reporting single-case designs in sport and exercise have used overt performance, a substantial proportion have used the client's own reports of their behaviours, thoughts and feelings. Kazdin (1978) suggested that a predominant focus on overt performance rather than on self-report can be traced back to the heritage of applied behaviour analysis. With humans we are interested in their behaviour, and what they say about their performance may also be of interest, but what they say and what they do might not relate, which affects the problems they want treated and how well their actual behaviour is altered after treatment (Kazdin 1982).

As we have discussed in detail in Chapter 3 there is an inherent problem in research with human participants. Both the participants and the observers are subject to response biases and sets. For instance, the client may respond in a socially desirable fashion or lie about how they are feeling before competition. These instances highlight how distorted one's view of performance could be. And the same is true of observers conducting behavioural assessment. Simply, when people are aware that others are assessing their behaviour, they distort what they say and what they do. If we are measuring anxiety, self-confidence or intrusive thoughts, self-report might be the only possible method of assessment. In sport and exercise settings, when the client is the only one with direct access to how she or he is feeling, for example, then self-report becomes the primary assessment modality. Indeed, many researchers in sport have assessed constructs such as self-efficacy, motivation and emotions using self-report (e.g., Barker and Jones 2008; Jones 2003). The client's private experience might be relevant to the problem identified and the prime reason for the client to seek treatment (Kazdin 1982).

Many studies in sport have used athlete self-monitoring. For example, McKenzie and Rushall (1974) used athlete self-monitoring to monitor laps swum during swimming practices. Hume, Martin, Gonzalez, Cracklen and Genthon (1985) used a self-monitoring feedback package to improve freestyle skating performance. Kirschenbaum, Owens and O'Connor (1998) used self-monitoring to improve and score the mental game in golf. Critchfield and Vargas (1991) replicated McKenzie and Rushall's original experiment in which swimmers were observed under four different conditions introduced sequentially: no intervention, instructions to swim, instructions to self-monitor and instructions to self-graph the self-monitored data. In contrast to McKenzie and Rushall's study, the coach's feedback was limited or absent to remove the coach as a confounding factor by prompting or praising the actions of the swimmer. Swimmers swam the greatest number of lengths when the experimenters introduced the self-monitoring condition. The authors explained that the self-monitoring procedure was sufficient to enhance swimming performance during practice because performance did not increase significantly when they introduced the self-graphing manipulation.

Performance profiling

Another behavioural recording technique employed by sport psychologists in professional practice is performance profiling – a technique that encourages athletes to identify qualities that they deem to be important to performance and then to rate themselves on each of these skills (Weston 2008). Performance profiling is a strategy used to uncover an athlete's perspective of his or her strengths and weaknesses (Butler and Hardy 1992). Many sport psychologists use this strategy to increase the client's volitional behaviour within a mental skills intervention. Butler (1989) devised performance profiling as an application of Kelly's (1955) personal construct theory (PCT) to sport psychology with a repertory grid used to help a sport performer develop a personal construct system. The repertory grid or performance profile allows the performer to plot those characteristics and qualities that are important to the performer rather than completing questionnaires set by the sport psychologist. This strategy typically involves three steps. First, the athlete is asked to identify all the characteristics and qualities of an elite performer in her sport. Next, the athlete evaluates her current level of mastery of each of those characteristics and qualities. Finally, those specific characteristics and qualities in which the athlete is deficient fulfil the target behaviours for improvement. Jones (1993) used performance profiling with an elite female racquet sport player who suffered with her temperament on court, becoming angry and frustrated in pressure situations. Performance profiling served three purposes in this study: (1) to help the sport psychologist to form an appropriate psychological intervention; (2) to maximize the performer's motivation to participate and adhere to the intervention; and (3) to monitor changes during the intervention.

Videotaping behaviours

Videotaping behaviour presents observers with a permanent record of that behaviour for observational analysis (Kendall, Hrycaiko, Martin and Kendall 1990; Tkachuk et al. 2003). This record can be observed after the performance to identify those behaviours of interest. Practitioners have used videotape analysis to develop sport skills (Boyer, Miltenberger, Batsche and Fogel 2009; Hazen, Johnstone, Martin and Srikameswaren 1990) and to recover lost skills (Collins et al. 1999). Tkachuk et al. (2003) suggested using videotape analysis to determine the components of effective and ineffective pre-competition or pre-performance routines. Researchers improve verbal and non-verbal behaviour assessment by using videotape to cue recall of verbal behaviour and emotions experienced during the performance (Schwartz and Garamoni 1986). Boyer et al. (2009) examined the effects of video modelling by experts with video feedback among four female competitive gymnasts (seven to ten years old) in a multiple-baseline design across behaviours. During the treatment, a gymnast performed a gymnastic skill and then watched a video replay of her performance. The gymnasts improved their performance across three gymnastics skills following exposure to the intervention.

Computer-assisted data collection

Data collection devices such as hand-held computers have been used in clinical psychology; however, this technique is not usually used in sport settings. Computer-assisted self-monitoring is worth exploring because it has been used successfully in research with obese clients who used hand-held computers to monitor weight, caloric intake, exercise, daily goals and goal attainment (Tkachuk et al. 2003).

Psychophysiological assessment

Psychophysiological responses have been assessed in single-case designs in sport and exercise. Psychophysiological responses directly reflect many problems of clinical significance or are highly correlated with the occurrence of such problems (Kazdin 1982). For example, it is important to assess autonomic arousal in disorders associated with anxiety. One can observe overt behavioural signs of arousal; however, physiological arousal can be assessed directly and presents a crucial component of arousal in its own right. Much of the impetus for psychophysiological assessment in single-case research has come from the emergence of biofeedback, in which the client is presented with information about his or her ongoing physiological processes. Assessment of psychophysiological responses in biofeedback research has encompassed diverse disorders and processes of cardiovascular, respiratory, gastrointestinal, genitourinary, musculoskeletal and other systems.

Some of the more commonly reported measures in single-case research include psychophysiological measures such as heart or pulse rate, blood pressure, skin temperature, blood volume, muscle tension and brain wave activity. Prapavessis et al. (1992) used a single-subject research design to test the effectiveness of a cognitive-behavioural intervention in reducing state anxiety and improving sport performance for a small-bore rifle shooter who suffered from high levels of competition-related anxiety. The authors gathered self-report, physiological and behavioural measures of baseline state anxiety during competition. Three separate physiological indicators of state anxiety were recorded: electromyographic responses (EMGs), electrocardiographic responses (ECGs) and urine samples to assess catecholamine (i.e., noradrenaline and adrenaline) concentrations. Following a six-week intervention including relaxation, thought stoppage, refocusing, coping statements and biofeedback, cognitive and somatic anxiety, gun vibration and urinary catecholamines decreased while self-confidence and performance increased from baseline to treatment.

Observations

If a sport psychologist is invited to work with a gymnast, he or she might choose to understand the behaviour of the gymnast by observing performance at training and competition (this is a similar situation to that outlined in the case study reported by Mace et al. 1987 in Chapter 1). In this example the observation is naturalistic because the psychologist is not intentionally intervening or structuring the situation for the client (Kazdin 1982). This direct observation as it occurs naturally in training and competition offers much information to understand the behaviour of the client (i.e., the gymnast). Although much information can be gleaned from these observations, at times the information that the sport psychologist is hoping to find is not apparent. For instance, how does this gymnast perform under pressure in a national competition? In this instance it might not be possible for the sport psychologist to see the gymnast in action under these conditions because of the low frequency of the behaviour or the unexpected conditions. If, however, the coach organized an artificial situation to observe the gymnast, it might be possible to assess the target behaviour. For instance, the coach might organize a simulated competition with background sound reflecting an audience and qualified judges to observe and judge the gymnast's performance on her floor routine. The advantage of this contrived condition is that information is now available that might not be available about the client during a typical training session. Without this set-up, it is possible that the coach or sport psychologist might not see a particular behaviour. Also, contrived situations provide consistent and standardized assessment conditions that can be observed over time (Kazdin 1982). Regrettably, this situation also means that the contrived situation might bear little relation to performance under naturalistic conditions. For instance, the communicative behaviour of a coach teaching young children sport skills can be assessed by setting up structured tasks for the children to perform and observing the coach's verbal and non-verbal behaviour. Under such conditions, however, the coach and children might behave in ways that are socially desirable, but not how they would behave under normal circumstances. However, a contrived situation might offer the only alternative to a naturalistic setting for the observer.

But naturalistic settings also have costs to bear. It might be too costly to observe behaviour over time in a naturalistic setting. To ensure reliability, these observations would require some inter-rater assessment and the assessment conditions might change with each occasion being observed. In an effort to deal with these challenges we can observe behaviour in a laboratory setting for convenience and standardization of assessment. If clients know that their behaviour is being observed, they often alter their behaviour and in certain conditions the sport psychologist must choose the correct strategy to account for any distorted behaviour. This challenges the observer to choose between obtrusive and unobtrusive assessment. Although a sport performer may be aware that a sport psychologist or coach is observing his behaviour, he might not know exactly which behaviour is being observed. If, however, the sport psychologist is observing a particular behaviour and the client is aware, he might alter his behaviour (the Hawthorne effect outlined in Chapter 3). Unobtrusive behavioural observations are rarely reported in sport and exercise studies. Ethically, it is problematic to observe behaviour and withhold information.

Whether we observe behaviour naturally or in contrived conditions, in laboratory settings with obtrusive or unobtrusive measures, humans are the observers (Kazdin 1982). Humans record behaviour at the training ground, at a competition venue or in the laboratory, and although they might be specially brought in to carry out the observations they might also be there already, for example a parent at a training session or a coach. Sometimes, automated devices may be used to record behaviour. Such a device might be used to record a response, and its duration or influence on subsequent performance. After calibration, the apparatus records the behaviour and the numerical output is used to understand behaviour. In sport, for example, a powerful technique to help a performer learn how to self-regulate arousal is biofeedback. Biofeedback is a technique that uses instruments to provide information about the state of selected biological functions that are not usually under voluntary control (Bar-Eli, Dreshman, Blumenstein and Weinstein 2002; Zaichkowsky and Takenaka 1993). Sport psychologists have used many biofeedback modalities such as EMG, skin temperature, galvanic skin response (GSR), heart rate and ECG. Bar-Eli et al. (2002) suggested using ideographic methods such as case studies and applied behaviour analysis because personality and situational variables help determine a performer's response to being assigned to a specific treatment condition.

Interobserver agreement

Interobserver agreement is the degree to which two or more independent observers report the same occurrences of an event after measuring the same event (Cooper et al. 2007). Humans, for the most part, observe the behaviour of others but they are fallible observers, even when they are well trained before the study (Morgan and Morgan 2009). And when a human observes behaviour, we cannot know the extent to which that observer's data reflect the behaviour of the person being observed. To address this issue and to maintain the integrity of the measurement process, researchers assign two observers to independently observe the behaviour of a client. When they have completed their assessment, they can determine whether their observations match. The researcher can calculate the measure of agreement between the observers, which is called interobserver agreement (Johnston and Pennypacker 2009).

This technique cannot impart information about accuracy or reliability because true values are required to assess accuracy and reliability and it depends upon comparing results of repeated observations of the same events (Johnston and Pennypacker 2009). When two observers agree, we only know that they agree about seeing a particular behaviour; however, we cannot know for sure that it actually happened. But scientific measurement means researchers make every effort to obtain the information properly, which means that each observer is trained to observe the participant, without obstructing the view or ability to hear other observers and also without knowing how the other observers are recording responses.

Interobserver agreement can be assessed using various methods. It can be calculated for frequency, duration and time sampling. Perhaps the simplest way to calculate interobserver agreement is to calculate the percentage agreement among the observers. Researchers also refer to the interobserver agreement as interobserver reliability and inter-rater reliability. For example, two observers might count the number of completed passes by a midfield player during the first quarter of a football game. The primary observer records seventeen completed passes, and the secondary observer records fifteen completed passes. By dividing the smaller number by the bigger number and then multiplying that number by 100 per cent, we can obtain the percentage agreement: $15/17 \times 100$ per cent $= 88$ per cent. In this example, however, this percentage does not explain whether the two observers agreed or disagreed on specific instances of behaviour. Boyer et al. (2009) examined the effects of combining video modelling by experts with video feedback among four female competitive gymnasts (seven to ten years old). Three target behaviours were assessed including a backward giant circle to handstand, a kip cast and a clear hip circle. Each skill had a twenty-eight-item checklist with each component scored as either correct or incorrect. The authors calculated the percentage of agreement by dividing the number of agreements by the number of agreements plus disagreements for the twenty-eight components of each skill.

Observers must also calculate the duration that they observe the target behaviour to ensure that they are observing for the same period of time; otherwise, checking the reliability of the observers' data is worthless. The duration represents the amount of time between the onset and the offset of the target behaviour (Morgan and Morgan 2009). Taking our example above, if the observers were calculating the number of passes completed by a midfielder in the second half of a football game and the primary observer reported forty-five minutes' duration but the secondary observer included injury time to record forty-eight minutes' duration, we would divide the smaller number by the bigger number and multiply by 100 per cent: $45/48 \times 100$ per cent $= 94$ per cent agreement between the observers.

Interval recording and time sampling add more dimensions to interobserver agreement. Rather than just calculating how often or for how long the behaviour occurred, the researcher must also calculate the percentage of intervals that observers agree that the behaviour did or did not occur. For example, if two observers record whether the behaviour occurred or did not occur – a dichotomous recording decision – we can calculate the interobserver agreement for these data by calculating the overall percentage of agreement across intervals. Four possible outcomes can emerge. First, the primary and secondary observers record a behaviour occurring, resulting in an agreement. Second, if both observers record a non-occurrence, this also represents an agreement. Third, if the primary observer records an occurrence but the secondary observer records a non-occurrence, this represents a disagreement. Finally, the primary observer might record a non-occurrence whereas the secondary observer might record an occurrence; this also represents a disagreement.

One difficulty that emerges is when neither observer records an instance of behaviour, which can happen with subtle behaviours, low rates of behaviour or brief intervals (Morgan and Morgan 2009). To address this issue, Cooper et al. (2007) suggested reporting three indices of agreement: (1) occurrences when the behaviour is observed in 30 per cent or fewer intervals; (2) non-occurrences only when behaviour is scored in 70 per cent or more intervals; and (3) occurrences and non-occurrences.

Many threats to accurate and reliable measurement emerge in single-case designs. Because humans are involved in measuring behaviour, instances of human error arise. At least three factors can account for human measurement error: poorly designed measurement systems, inadequate observer training and observer expectations of the data (Cooper et al. 2007). Poorly designed measurement systems reduce the accuracy and reliability of records of the target behaviour. If we consider the preceding section, we might record more than one individual or behaviour, as well as the duration of observation periods and the observation intervals. Together, these affect the quality of measurement because of their complexity. Researchers, where possible, should reduce the complexity of measurement and practise more during observer training to ensure the observation procedure is mastered. Collecting trustworthy data is only possible if observers are chosen carefully and trained to code target behaviour(s) properly. They must understand the distinction between the occurrence and the non-occurence of the target behaviour. Observers may succumb to observer drift when they alter, often innocently, how they apply a measurement system. In other words, the observer understands the original definition of the target behaviour but shifts that understanding to include or exclude particular occurrences of the target behaviour. Researchers can minimize observer drift with occasional sessions to retrain the observer and to provide feedback on the accuracy and reliability of measurement. Finally, if an observer holds specific expectations of the data, he or she might record data that fulfil that expectation. For example, if an observer is recording the effect of positive reinforcement on a child's on-task behaviour, he or she might record more instances of that behaviour. Naïve observers, unaware of the study's purpose, could be used to minimize this effect. But observers are also aware that others (e.g., researcher, secondary observer) are evaluating the data they collect, known as observer reactivity. Not only do participants alter their behaviour when they are observed but also the observers alter their own behaviour. To overcome this issue, it is better to monitor observers discreetly and, where possible, to separate multiple observers by distance or partition (Cooper et al. 2007).

Summary

Behavioural interventions typically aim to enhance performance or skill acquisition on the one hand, or produce helpful psychosocial outcomes such as increasing sport enjoyment or self-esteem and reducing dropout and performance anxiety on the other (Smith and Smoll 1996; Smith, Smoll and Christensen 1996). Although we might work to overcome behavioural deficits or decrease behavioural excesses, small changes in the target behaviour might be meaningful. For an elite athlete, an improvement in performance, however slight, might have dramatic effects on that athlete's competitive success (Smith and Smoll 1996). Therefore, assessing behaviour demands that researchers and practitioners fastidiously measure behaviour. We have numerous tools available to measure behaviour obtrusively or unobtrusively but we must ensure that we rigorously check that each observer is accurately recording the target behaviour in the behaviour change programme. In the following chapters we explore some of the common designs of single-case research.

Key points

* Behavioural assessment represents an essential element in the behaviour change programme in sport and exercise.
* Researchers and practitioners have numerous techniques available to them to measure behaviour accurately.
* Researchers and practitioners must ensure that measuring instruments provide accurate and reliable measures of the target behaviour under investigation.
* Multiple observers should measure the target behaviour and interobserver agreement should be reported in the single-case study.

Guided study

Your task in this chapter is to locate from journals three studies using a single-case research design and explain the type of behavioural assessment used in each study. You'll find examples in the *Journal of Applied Behavioral Analysis*, *The Sport Psychologist*, *Psychology of Sport and Exercise* and the *Journal of Applied Sport Psychology*. Read the questions below first before reading the studies to find the answers. For each study:

* What type of behavioural assessment was used?
* Was the behavioural assessment tool suitable for the aims of the study?
* If more than one person observed the target variable, was the inter-observer agreement reported?
* Did any issues arise with the definition of the target variable?
* What challenges were reported in measuring the target variable?

5

THE WITHDRAWAL DESIGN IN SPORT AND EXERCISE

In this chapter, we will:

- outline the rationale for withdrawal designs in sport and exercise;
- outline variations of the withdrawal design;
- provide guidance on using this design in applied sport and exercise contexts.

CASE EXAMPLE

Lucy is a sixteen-year-old junior golfer who has experienced a large amount of success in her junior career so far. However, during recent tournaments she has noticed her focus during shots often drifts and she has a tendency to become distracted by thoughts and objects in the immediate environment. For example, when standing on the tee box where a water hazard is in view her focus is drawn to the hazard and not to cues relevant to the successful execution of the shot. The sport psychologist working with Lucy decides to spend some time walking the course with her during tournaments to gain an insight into her pre-shot preparation. He concludes that her pre-shot approach is inconsistent in both routine and duration. Furthermore, he ascertains that to perform at a higher level her attentional focus will need to be improved.

Introduction and basic rationale for the design

So far in this book we have outlined the fundamental rationale, features and benefits of single-case methods for sport and exercise settings. Alongside this background information, researchers and practitioners should understand the design options under the single-case umbrella. In more traditional research methods, many design options cater for situations that arise in applied behavioural science research (see Clark-Carter 2009). Single-case research methods also contain many design options for the same reasons. Therefore the following chapters sketch the main designs available in single-case research. However, this chapter describes a basic design option, notably the withdrawal or reversal, or A–B–A, design (Kazdin 1982). The chapter begins with an overview of the design and examples from the sport and exercise literature. Next we consider variations of the standard withdrawal design (e.g., A–B–A–B design) and provide further illustrations from the literature. The chapter concludes with an evaluation of the design including its strengths and limitations and guidance for scientists and practitioners.

The withdrawal design is a basic single-case design that involves first presenting and then removing an independent variable (i.e., an intervention or treatment) from a participant or participant group (Kazdin 1982). The withdrawal design is also referred to as an A–B–A or a reversal design because of the sequence of experimental conditions exclusive to this design. To illustrate, the design typically comprises the following sequence: non-treatment (A) phase, treatment (B) phase, non-treatment (A) phase. Because of this sequence the design is regarded as a robust and powerful procedure for assessing the effects of an independent variable (i.e., intervention or treatment) on target variables (e.g., exercise adherence, coaching instruction) in applied research. The principal logic of the withdrawal design (and other single-case variations) is based on determining or drawing causal inference, for example allowing a researcher or practitioner to ascertain if an intervention brought about change in a targeted behaviour (Kazdin 1982; Kinugasa et al. 2004; Kratochwill et al. 1984; Morgan and Morgan 2009).

All scientific research begins with observation, and in the behavioural sciences observation is a key element of its research methodology. Once important decisions have been made about selecting and measuring target variables (e.g., behaviour and performance), observation and data collection can begin. The withdrawal design (like other single-case variations) contains a number of fundamental components. First, observation of pre-treatment target variables and responses takes place in a baseline phase (A). Typically, the baseline phase should be a stable, representative picture of the behaviour of the targeted variable(s) and should indicate a participant's 'natural state' before treatment or intervention. It is particularly important that the baseline displays a level of consistency across data points because one should be able to predict what the variables would be like in the future if an intervention was not implemented (Kazdin 1982). A potential caveat to the collection of baseline data arises when variables are observed continually. Over time, fluctuations or small deviations can be expected in the data. Indeed, variables cannot be expected to remain entirely stable and some variables (e.g., behaviours) are likely to be more variable than others. To allow for comparison between baseline and post-treatment data, it is essential that the amount of variability in the observed variable is minimal and that there are no apparent substantial upwards or downwards trends in baseline data before the intervention is implemented (Morgan and Morgan 2009).

Stability in data (or 'steady state') is a critical element of most single-case designs because it allows one to compare variables (e.g., behaviour) at baseline with variables following a treatment. From this comparison it is possible to draw conclusions about intervention effectiveness. In contrast, if variables display signs of inconsistency (i.e., upwards and downwards trends) in baseline data (i.e., when the intervention is not present) then one's ability to interpret any intervention effect is likely to be compromised. In essence, the steady state reflects a control phase and is therefore a pivotal component of most single-case designs. In addition to the stability of baseline data, one must also be aware of the natural cycles and fluctuations in behaviour that occur as a consequence of physiological (e.g., illness) and/or environment factors (e.g., a lack of sleep in hot weather). This behavioural cyclicity is a naturally occurring phenomenon and is suggested not to be a confounding variable as long as baselines are long enough to cater for such variation (Bloom et al. 2009). Although efforts have been made to quantify effective baseline lengths (e.g., Callow and Waters 2005; Ottenbacher 1986) to account for steady state and behaviour cyclicity, the collection of baseline data depends on practical, ethical and logistical constraints – as we will discover in the following chapters. In summary, the baseline allows for comparison with behaviours or responses once an intervention is presented.

The second feature of withdrawal designs is that, following collection of a steady and consistent baseline (where ethically and logistically possible), the manipulation of the independent variable (i.e., presentation of an intervention) takes place (B). Typically, manipulation of the independent variable occurs through an intervention. By convention, the baseline and intervention phases are suggested to have equivalent intervals (Barlow and Hersen 1984; Cooper et al. 2007; Kazdin 1994). For example, if baseline data are collected across eight trials lasting four weeks then the intervention phase should last the same length of time. Through the presentation of this intervention it is possible to manipulate the dependent variables. Indeed, changes in the dependent variables following an intervention allow conclusions to be drawn about intervention effectiveness. To illustrate, following the presentation of the intervention, data are typically compared using graphical or statistical methods (see Chapters 3 and 9). Hypothetical data to illustrate this comparison are provided in Figure 5.1. In essence, this figure highlights the baseline phase, during which psychometric attention scores were collected before nine rounds of golf; the intervention phase, demonstrated with the dashed line; and post-intervention data, collected before nine rounds of golf.

From this figure you will notice that the graph is split into two halves separated by a vertical line indicating when the intervention was presented. This

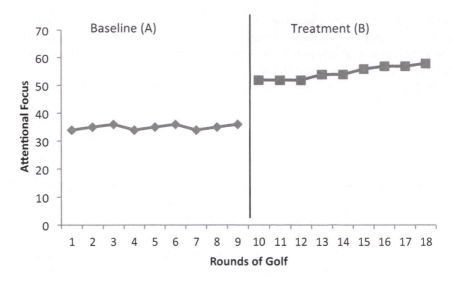

FIGURE 5.1 The A–B phase change.

presentation is a common method of reporting single-case data (for a more in-depth discussion see Chapter 9). Figure 5.1 also demonstrates a common single-case variation in the form of the A–B design. Typically, this design involves the collection of baseline data (A) on a target behaviour followed by data collection after the intervention (B). Both sets of data are then compared to determine intervention effectiveness. An example from sport demonstrates an A–B design. As mentioned in Chapter 1, Barker and Jones (2008) reported the effects of a hypnosis intervention on a professional soccer player who demonstrated low self-efficacy and a negative mood state relative to his soccer performance. Eight baseline (A phase) and eight post-intervention (B phase) data points were collected by means of a Soccer Self-Efficacy Questionnaire (SSEQ) that consisted of ten items relating to good soccer performance, the Positive and Negative Affect Schedule (PANAS; Watson, Clarke and Tellegen 1988) and a Soccer Performance Measure (SPM). The intervention programme consisted of eight hypnosis sessions. These sessions comprised the presentation of ego-strengthening suggestions. Both visual and statistical analysis revealed substantial increases in self-efficacy, positive affect and soccer performance, as well as a substantial decrease in negative affect, over the course of the intervention. Of course, with an A–B design it is possible that any observed differences may be the consequence of natural development and not because of the intervention. Therefore the withdrawal design is considered a more robust design for drawing causal inferences about intervention effectiveness (Lavallee, Williams and Jones 2008).

The final feature of the withdrawal design is the return to baseline, or non-treatment condition (A), after a treatment phase. The rationale for this reversal is to determine if a certain behaviour change was due to the intervention and not to some other variable: withdrawing the intervention should return behaviour to baseline levels. Accordingly, the reversal phase (A) is a check of the effect of an intervention by allowing researchers and practitioners to make a judgement about causal inference. For example, the A–B–A design permits this at two levels: first with the initial presentation of the intervention and second when the intervention is removed. Figure 5.2 presents an example of the A–B–A design in which it is evident that the intervention has brought about a change in the targeted behaviour. Indeed, this figure demonstrates the clear differences in attentional focus between baseline, treatment and withdrawal phases; one observes that without the intervention attentional focus is at a lower level.

Because drawing inferences in science depends largely on reducing or eliminating confounding factors, and/or rival explanations of the data, researchers and practitioners involved in applied research must be certain that their interventions have brought about any observed changes in behaviour (Bryan 1987). Therefore, the structure of the A–B–A design provides a suitable platform from which to make causal inferences about intervention effectiveness, particularly when baseline levels return to baseline following an intervention. Finally, highlighting that change was due only to an intervention establishes a study's internal validity. When a researcher can rule out extraneous variables as a potential explanation for changes in target variables, confidence is increased in the effectiveness of the intervention (Smith 1988).

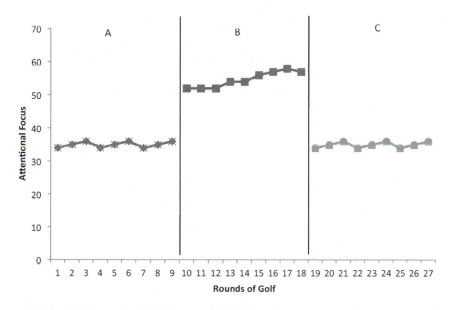

FIGURE 5.2 The withdrawal design.

You may recall our case study, Lucy, from earlier in the chapter. She was a junior golfer with limited attentional control. The sport psychologist working with her decided to use a behaviour intervention (i.e., the development of a pre-performance routine; PPR) to enhance her attentional focus. To determine the effect of the PPR, the psychologist used a withdrawal design. Initially, a baseline was established with data collected on Lucy's pre-shot thoughts across eight competitive rounds. Following the baseline a PPR was developed for Lucy. After a two-week intensive practice of the PPR she began to use the routine in tournament play. For eight competitive rounds the psychologist again monitored her pre-shot thoughts. Following these rounds the psychologist informed Lucy that she should discontinue her use of the PPR despite her thoughts and performances improving substantially from baseline. Reluctantly, Lucy withdrew her use of the PPR so that data could be collected for a further eight rounds. Data from this phase indicated that her thoughts and performances had returned to baseline, thus supporting conclusions about the effectiveness of the PPR.

Although this example reveals how the A–B–A design can provide researchers with clear evidence about the effects of an intervention, it does pose a number of problems for the participant involved – particularly as Lucy was required to relinquish a strategy that brought about profitable gains. This dilemma and other issues relating to the use of the withdrawal design in applied research contexts are discussed later in the chapter.

Treatment integrity

In Chapter 3 we focused on the importance in single-case research of accurately measuring the dependent variables of the targeted behaviour or outcome. In addition, it is important to describe adequately the independent variables (i.e., intervention) used within applied practice and research (Morgan and Morgan 2009). The term 'treatment integrity' refers to the researcher's responsibility to describe in specific detail the intervention and procedures within a study so that other practitioners and researchers can consistently deliver and replicate similar interventions on other samples. Treatment integrity is important as it provides information on how an intervention has been operationalized and optimized. For example, information about the time and effort taken to deliver an intervention is important for researchers and practitioners wishing to replicate a study. Further, the extent to which sport and exercise researchers have considered treatment integrity is scant in comparison with the level of detail presented on the measurement of dependent variables in published mainstream applied research (e.g., McDougall, Skouge, Farrell and Hoff 2006; Perepletchikova and Kazdin 2005). Thus, treatment integrity is an issue that sport and exercise researchers and practitioners should consider when publishing applied research to allow for study replication. To illustrate, Barker and Jones (2008) is a good example of this because the hypnosis scripts used in the intervention were included in the published manuscript.

The A–B–A (withdrawal) design in sport and exercise: illustrations

The basic rationale for the A–B–A (withdrawal design) has been outlined in the previous section. In this section we outline two examples of this approach from the sport and exercise literature.

The first illustration of an A–B–A design comes from a study by Lerner, Ostrow, Yura and Etzel (1996) who investigated the effects of goal-setting and imagery programmes, as well as a combined goal-setting and imagery training programme, on free-throw performance among female collegiate basketball players over the course of an entire season. Their design consisted of an A–B–A (withdrawal) multiple-baseline design. Twelve players were randomly assigned to one of three interventions: (1) goal-setting ($n = 4$), (2) imagery ($n = 4$) or (3) goal-setting and imagery ($n = 4$). During baseline (A) each basketball player shot twenty free throws at each session. Each of the sessions took place on the basketball court during non-competitive, practice conditions. Because the study used a multiple-baseline approach (discussed further in Chapter 6), after non-competitive free-throw performance reached a stable rate for one individual in each of the three groups, the intervention was applied to that individual while baseline conditions continued for the other participants. The intervention was staggered across the basketball season. The researchers decided that stability in baseline was determined by observing at least six consecutive sessions in which individual performance did not deviate by more than two free-throw shots. One-third of the participants were exposed to a goal-setting intervention (B) following baseline. The goal-setting intervention consisted of teaching each player how to set effective goals according to guidelines presented in previous research (e.g., Burton 1989; Gould 1993). Following this goal-setting intervention, the players were asked to set a performance goal prior to shooting at each session. The one-third of participants who were assigned to the imagery group received training (B) consisting of imagery tapes and education (Burton 1989). Each imagery session was held once per day and lasted for approximately fifteen minutes, prior to free-throw performance. Participants listened to their imagery tape and then attempted twenty free throws under non-competitive conditions. Finally, one-third of participants received both goal-setting and imagery training (B), which consisted of listening to an imagery tape (similar to that used in the imagery group), setting a performance goal (based on similar guidelines as presented in the goal-setting group) and then attempting twenty free-throws. Every participant had ten intervention sessions. Following the intervention phase, a second baseline phase (A; withdrawal phase) was instigated for ten sessions, in which each player took twenty free throws per session. Importantly, to monitor the effects of withdrawing the interventions, the participants were instructed not to employ their goal-setting or imagery strategies during this second baseline. Data collected during each of the study's sessions revealed that free-throw performance improved for three participants in the goal-setting programme and for one participant in the goal-setting and imagery programme, whereas performance for three participants in the imagery programme decreased (see Figure 5.3).

The second example of a withdrawal design (i.e., A–B–A) comes from research by Pates, Maynard and Westbury (2001) who investigated the effects of hypnosis on basketball set and jump performance in three male collegiate basketball players. Specifically, the experimental design consisted of a baseline where data on set and jump performance were collected on each participant

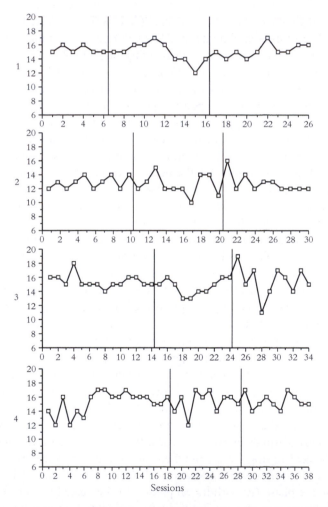

FIGURE 5.3 Free-throw performance for imagery participants. Adapted with permission from B. S. Lerner, A. C. Ostrow, M. Yura and E. F. Etzel (1996) The effects of goal-setting and imagery training programmes on the free-throw performance of female collegiate basketball players. *The Sport Psychologist, 10,* 382–397.

for four weeks (i.e., eight trials). Once stable baselines had been determined, the treatment (hypnosis intervention) was introduced and data again measured across approximately four weeks (i.e., eight trials). Following withdrawal of the intervention, the baseline phase was re-instated. This second baseline once again involved eight trials over four weeks. In addition, throughout the study interview data were collected after each trial to monitor participants' internal experience (Wollman 1986). The intervention consisted of the use of hypnosis. Specifically, hypnosis training comprised four stages: relaxation, hypnotic induction, hypnotic regression and trigger control. Following the training, participants committed themselves to practice of the techniques and this was facilitated by the daily use of a hypnosis audio tape (containing the training method) over a seven-day period. After the training period, players began the intervention phase and were instructed to use their trigger word each time they performed a jump or set shot. Before the second baseline, the audio tapes were retrieved, and instructions given to not use the triggers during the jump and set performance trials. The results indicated that all three participants increased their mean jump and set shooting performance from baseline to intervention, with all three returning to baseline levels in the withdrawal phase (see Figure 5.4). In addition, interview data regarding participants' internal experience of the study indicated that they felt that the intervention had increased sensations that they associated with peak performance.

Overall, the two preceding examples highlight how the use of an A–B–A design (using a small *n* and the rigorous evaluation of individual behaviour change and treatment effects) has allowed the researchers to ascertain who did or did not respond to an intervention or who responded in erratic fashion. This type of intervention information would typically not be available in traditional between-group comparisons (Bryan 1987; Wollman 1986).

Interim summary

The A–B–A (withdrawal) design is a common single-case research design used within mainstream applied behavioural research, but is less prevalent in the sport and exercise literature. The withdrawal design may be an undesirable choice for individuals involved in sport and exercise because reversing the gains made in the initial treatment phase may not meet their performance demands (Bryan 1987). The premise of the design is intra-subject replication to evaluate the effectiveness of an intervention. The initial baseline phase (A) is used to establish the natural occurrence of a targeted behaviour to exposure to an intervention. Following stabilization of baseline behaviours, an intervention phase (B) is then implemented, and changes in the targeted behaviour are compared with baseline. Finally, a return to baseline (A) permits the researcher and/or practitioner to establish if observed changes in behaviour were a result of the intervention and not the result of an extraneous variable (Morgan and Morgan 2009). The following sections illustrate the most common variations of

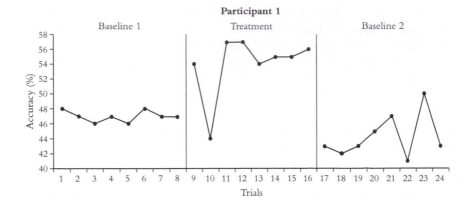

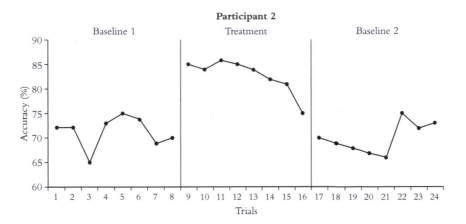

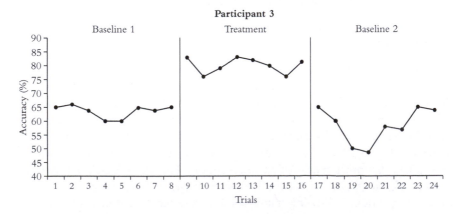

FIGURE 5.4 Set-shooting performance accuracy for participants 1, 2, and 3. Adapted from J. Pates, I. Maynard and T. Westbury (1996) An investigation into the effects of hypnosis on basketball performance. *Journal of Applied Sport Psychology, 13*, 84–102 (Taylor & Francis Ltd, http://www.informaworld. com) by permission of the publisher.

the withdrawal design used in applied practice and research and how these can be applied to sport- and exercise-related individuals and settings.

Design variations

The A–B–A–B design

The A–B–A–B design examines the effects of an intervention by alternating the baseline condition (A) with the intervention condition (B). The A and B phases are repeated to complete four phases of the withdrawal variation, making this a stronger approach than the A–B–A method (Kazdin 1982). Intervention effectiveness is determined if target variables (e.g., performance) improve during the first intervention phase, revert to or approach original baseline levels when the intervention is withdrawn, and improve when treatment is re-introduced in the second intervention phase (Kazdin 1982; Kratochwill et al. 1984). Figure 5.5 illustrates hypothetical data for an A–B–A–B design. In the baseline phase, the level of the target variable(s) is assessed (depicted by the solid line) and then this line can be projected to predict the level of the variable(s) (dashed line). Accordingly, when a projection can be made with a level of confidence, the intervention (B) is implemented. The data in the intervention phase describe current behaviour and predict behaviour in the future if the intervention were not implemented (or had no effect). In addition, the researcher or practitioner can assess whether behaviour during the intervention phase (B, solid line) actually deviates from the projected level of baseline (B, dashed line). If behaviour does deviate in this

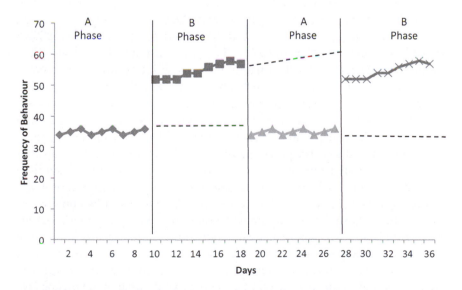

FIGURE 5.5 The A–B–A–B design.

first intervention phase, then this gives an indication of change as a consequence of the intervention. However, after only one A–B phase change it is difficult to draw causal inferences given that extraneous factors may have contributed to the change. Therefore, single-case studies that fit the A–B–A–B design extend to four or more phases to provide certainty about the effect of an intervention on the targeted variable(s). The third phase comprises withdrawing the intervention and reverting to baseline. According to Kazdin (1982) this second baseline (A phase) has three purposes: to describe current behaviour, predict future behaviour and test the level of behaviour predicted from the previous phase as outlined by the dashed line in the second A phase. In the final phase, the intervention is restored. This phase serves the same purpose as the previous phase: to describe behaviour, to explore whether performance deviates from the projected level of the previous phase and to explore whether performance is the same as predicted from the previous intervention phase (Kazdin 1994).

Overall, the A–B–A–B design consists of making and testing predictions about behaviour under different conditions (i.e., phases). Data from the four phases provide information about present behaviour, predict probable future behaviour and assess whether predictions were accurate. This variation provides an opportunity to repeatedly assess the effectiveness of an intervention on behaviour, thus enhancing internal validity (Kratochwill et al. 1984).

The A–B–A–B design in sport and exercise: illustrations

In the previous section, the major tenets of the A–B–A–B design were presented. What follows are examples of this design from research in sport and exercise settings. The A–B–A–B design has been used more extensively in sport and exercise settings in comparison with the standard withdrawal design described earlier (e.g., Allison and Ayllon 1980; Anderson and Kirkpatrick 2002; Barrett 2005; Heyman 1987; Hume et al. 1985). To illustrate, Hume et al. (1985) examined the effects of a self-management strategy intervention for improving practice performance in young figure skaters. For the three participants involved in the study, baseline performance (i.e., the total number of elements attempted in each training session) was monitored across each training session (A). Following baseline, an intervention consisting of a self-management package was introduced to participants one and two after eleven baseline measures, and participant 3 after thirteen measures (B). The intervention was then used by the participants for between five and seven training sessions before it was removed, reversing back to baseline conditions (A). This short baseline condition was then followed by the re-introduction of the self-management package (B). Data indicated that when the treatment was first introduced an immediate change in training performance was highlighted across all of the participants. To ascertain whether this effect was due to the intervention or an uncontrolled extraneous variable, the intervention was withdrawn. In each of the participants it was evident that performance returned to baseline levels. When the treatment was re-introduced in the final phase, performance immediately improved to pre-withdrawal levels, further illustrating the effectiveness of the intervention and reducing the likelihood of an extraneous variable causing the effect.

A study by Anderson and Kirkpatrick (2002) explored the effects of a behavioural treatment package on the performance (i.e., number of correct relay tags) of inline roller speed skaters using a multiple-baseline A–B–A–B design. The first phase included baselines (A) with staggered interventions (B) for three skaters. The intervention package consisted of verbal praise following correct tags, visual feedback of performance data and instruction for improving performance. The second phase took place six months later because treatment effects were not maintained. In this phase baseline was re-established (A) and the same intervention as described in phase one was re-instated, albeit simultaneously this time (B). One additional skater was introduced as a replication of the initial findings for the other three skaters. Data as highlighted in Figure 5.6 indicate that an immediate change in correct tags did occur for each of the skaters each time that the intervention was presented, although performance is somewhat variable across the treatment phases. Indeed, with such variability in performance it is difficult to ascertain that the intervention has been effective in this setting. The six-month gap between phases could have influenced this variability.

Finally, a study by Heyman (1987) revealed how a planned A–B–A–B design with an eighteen-year-old amateur boxer suffering from debilitating anxiety had to be modified to fit his needs and situation. Specifically, the coach and boxer could not wait for a lengthy baseline to be established because of the 'crisis' nature of the situation. The measures used in the study consisted of the number of punches thrown during each round, coach ratings of the boxer's offence and defence after each round, and self-reported anxiety ratings and perceptions of offence and defence after each round. Observations of the boxer took place in three up-and-coming events. First, two weeks following the initial consultations, a regional boxing competition was to be held that would allow the collection of baseline data. Second, two months after the regional event, a tri-team match was to take place in which the boxer would have two opponents, and which would allow for further data collection as well as attempting an intervention in one fight and not the other. Finally, some three months after the tri-match, the state competition was held and here data were collected with the intervention being used in all fights. Because of the 'crisis' situation and the sequence of forthcoming competition events, the planned A–B–A–B design had to be modified (Hersen and Barlow 1976). Therefore, in the study, baseline data were collected during the A_1 phase (the regional boxing match). In the second phase B_1 (the tri-team match competition), the intervention was to be implemented in the first fight, and then withdrawn in the second fight (phase three; A_2). In the final phase, the intervention was re-introduced (B_2). Indeed, despite the obvious look of an A–B–A–B design, the observations at baseline and throughout the study are not as lengthy as one would normally associate with

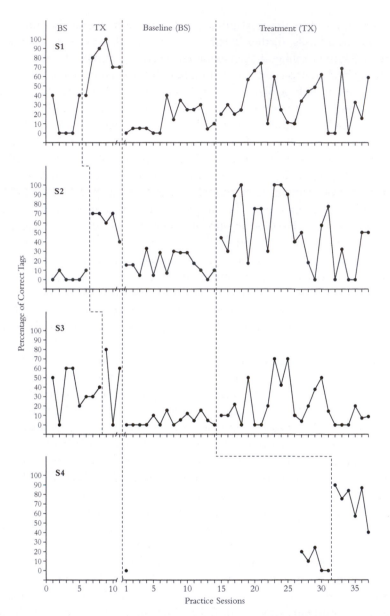

FIGURE 5.6 The percentage of trials in which relay tags were executed correctly as a function of baseline and behavioural intervention conditions for four skaters. The first A–B phase is shown in sessions 1–11. The second phase began approximately six months following the end of the first intervention. These data are presented after the break in the abscissa and are numbered 1–37. Adapted with permission from G. Anderson and M. A. Anderson (2002) Variable effects of a behavioral treatment package on the performance of inline roller speed skaters. *Journal of Applied Behavior Analysis, 35*, 195–198.

this type of design (Kazdin 1982). Nevertheless, it is important to recognize that the modification of the initial design was due in part to the needs of the coach and the boxer in not being able to wait for baseline to be established. The intervention used with the boxer comprised hypnotic procedures initially and then systematic desensitization. Three hypnosis sessions lasting around thirty minutes were used, with three hourly sessions a week for six weeks constituting the desensitization. Interestingly, as the tri-team competition approached the boxer became increasingly uncomfortable with first using and then discontinuing the intervention as he wanted to use it in both fights. This example therefore further highlights the ethical issues surrounding treatment withdrawal in applied research (Hersen and Barlow 1976). Overall, data collected across the study revealed that the intervention package seemed to have facilitated an improvement in the boxer's performance (i.e., number of punches thrown, defence and offence), and his anxiety levels, although the failure to establish multiple data points across the study perhaps limits the drawing of causal inference in this case. In summary, this study, although not a true A–B–A–B design (because of the A and B phases being separated by one fight each and with no stability in baseline or other phases), highlights how single-case designs can and do have to be adapted when used in applied research. Heyman did not have the opportunity to collect a lengthier baseline because of the time constraints imposed by the demands of the coach and boxer. In a situation such as this, one alternative may have been to use a probe design as outlined in Chapter 6, which does not carry the same baseline requirements as the A–B–A–B design for determining intervention effectiveness.

In this section, examples of the A–B–A–B design in sport and exercise settings have been illustrated in both research and applied contexts. The seminal work of Kazdin (1982) and Cooper et al. (2007) outlines a number of variations of the A–B–A–B design that cater for a variety of needs and circumstances. The following sections report some of the variations that may be pertinent to researchers and practitioners within sport and exercise settings.

The reversal phase

Although the withdrawal design relies on a return to baseline conditions to ascertain intervention effectiveness, there are other ways to show a relationship between behaviour and intervention using a withdrawal design (e.g., Goetz, Holmberg and LeBlanc 1975). One alternative is to administer consequences non-contingently. For example, during an intervention phase (B), a coach may deliver positive encouragement to alter an athlete's behaviour (e.g., carrying the ball out of defence). However, rather than withdrawing the positive encouragement to return to baseline, the coach may continue to provide the positive encouragement, but deliver it non-contingently, or independently of the athlete's behaviour. Moreover, this procedure is used to show that it is not the event (i.e., positive encouragement) that effects behaviour change but the relationship between the event and the behaviour. Indeed, non-contingent reinforcement should lead to a return of behaviour to baseline levels (Kazdin 1982). Non-contingent delivery can occur in other ways. For example, reinforcements of a specific behaviour (e.g., motivational instruction from a personal trainer) can be provided on the basis of elapsed time during a session (e.g., fifteen-minute intervals during a training session) rather than on an indiscriminate or a targeted basis. This form of delivery is likely to facilitate a return to baseline because the intervention is not being paired specifically with the targeted behaviour. Another variation of the reversal phase is to continue contingent consequences but to alter behaviours that are associated with the consequences. To illustrate, if an intervention comprises reinforcing certain aspects of behaviour (e.g., positive body language following an unforced error) the reversal phase can consist of reinforcing all behaviours except the one that was reinforced during the intervention (e.g., making passing shots, successful first serves). The procedure for doing so is called differential reinforcement of other behaviour (or DRO schedule). To illustrate, in an exercise class, praise on a DRO schedule may take place whenever exercisers are not working at a hard-enough intensity. The DRO schedule for showing a reversal of behaviour is used to demonstrate that the relationship between the target behaviour and the consequences rather than administration of the consequences accounts for behaviour change (Kazdin 1982). For example, Rowbury, Baer and Baer (1976) provided behaviour-problem school children with praise and tokens that could be exchanged for playtime. These rewards were presented for completing standard pre-academic tasks. A DRO schedule was used in the reversal phase in which tokens were given for just sitting around rather than for completing tasks. Under the DRO format, children completed fewer tasks than had been completed previously, thus the DRO served as a return to baseline or non-contingent delivery of consequences.

The order of phases

As previously outlined in this chapter, the A–B–A–B design typically begins with a baseline; however, a variation pertinent to the context of sport and exercise is when the design begins with an intervention (B phase). For example, circumstances (as Heyman found) may require an intervention to be administered immediately (e.g., a soccer player behaving aggressively in training, or being sent off following an on-field confrontation with a teammate), thus leaving no opportunity for baseline to be collected. In addition, starting a design with an intervention may also be appropriate when baseline levels are obvious because the behaviour may not have occurred (e.g., regular attendance at an exercise class for a new exerciser). In this situation the rationale behind a baseline lacks substance. Accordingly, in such situations, as outlined above, it is suggested to start a design with an intervention and then continue as a B–A–B–A design or when circumstances dictate a B–A–B design. Figure 5.7 provides a hypothetical example of this approach. This figure demonstrates how the intervention (i.e., praise), when presented in the first and third phases, leads to a higher frequency of the targeted behaviour compared with when the intervention is reversed in the second and fourth phases. The logic behind this approach is the same as in the A–B–A–B variation in that drawing inferences about intervention effectiveness is dependent on patterns of behaviour across the alternating phases (Cooper et al. 2007).

In summary, the B–A–B–A or B–A–B variations lend themselves particularly well to 'crisis' interventions when the gathering of stable baseline is not feasible in certain sport and exercise situations, and/or when the need for a baseline is unjustified or the pattern of baseline target variable(s) is obvious.

The number of phases

One of the main characteristics of the A–B–A–B design is that four phases are often used to determine intervention effectiveness. However, several options exist in relation to the number of phases required. To this end, Kazdin (1982) contended that, as a minimum, the withdrawal design must include *at least three phases* as either an A–B–A or a B–A–B format, as less than three affects the internal validity of the design. In addition, it is also possible to increase the number of the phases so that intervention effects are continuously demonstrated or when different interventions are included. Indeed, the use of an A–B–A–B–A–B design may be particularly useful in such circumstances.

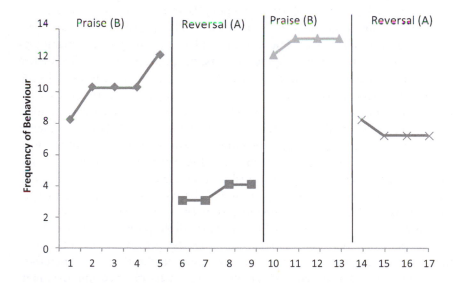

FIGURE 5.7 The B–A–B–A design.

Multiple interventions

Typically, the A–B–A–B design explores the effects of one intervention on target variables. However, the withdrawal design can also be varied depending on the number of interventions included in the design. For example, a sport psychologist may wish to use a multi-modal intervention comprising self-talk and imagery with a participant to reduce their anxiety. In this situation the separate interventions (B and C) are included in the same design. The multiple interventions variation is appropriate when one intervention does not work or when one wishes to examine the relative effectiveness of two separate interventions. In this context the interventions (B and C) are administered at different points in the design and are represented by an A–B–C–B–C–A or an A–B–C–A–B–C design (Kazdin 1978; Kratochwill et al. 1984). To illustrate, Messagno, Marchant and Morris (2008) investigated the effects of a pre-performance routine (PPR) on 'choking' in three ten-pin bowlers. Initially, eighty-eight experienced ten-pin bowlers completed a series of psychological inventories as a means of screening for 'choking-susceptible' participants. From this screening, three bowlers met 'choking-susceptible' criteria and were chosen for the study. The study adopted an A–B–A–C design in which manipulations of 'low pressure' and 'high pressure' occurred in the B and C phases respectively. The four phases included a first baseline (A_1), first pressure (B_1), second baseline (A_2) and intervention with pressure (C_1, referred to as B_2 by the authors) phase, and were scheduled separately over four weeks. Performance was measured by determining absolute error, in centimetres, from the centre of the target to the centre of the ball track on each shot. Testing commenced (A_1 phase) with participants completing sixty ten-pin bowling shots with one-minute rest periods separating each ten shots (trial block). Before the B_1 phase, participants were briefed about the pressure manipulation. This phase followed the same procedure as in the A_1 phase but with the addition of the pressure manipulation, which consisted of videotaping all shots, the presence of a small audience and financial incentives. During the A_2 phase the same procedures as in the A_1 baseline resumed. Before the start of the C_1 (B_2) phase, participants were instructed about the PPR. The PPR for each bowler included modification of arousal, behavioural steps, attention control and cue words (see Boutcher 1990). During the C_1 (B_2) phase, the same procedures as in the B_1 phase were used along with each participant using the PPR. Split-middle analyses (White 1974, 2005) across the three participants' data revealed improved bowling accuracy when using the PPR in comparison with bowling without a PPR. Indeed, data as illustrated in Figure 5.8 support this increase in bowling accuracy under high pressure with the use of a PPR. Despite these positive data, it is likely that participants were already desensitized to the pressure manipulation in the C_1 phase (B_2) because of exposure to pressure in the B_1 phase. Therefore, the desensitization may have contributed to the performance improvement.

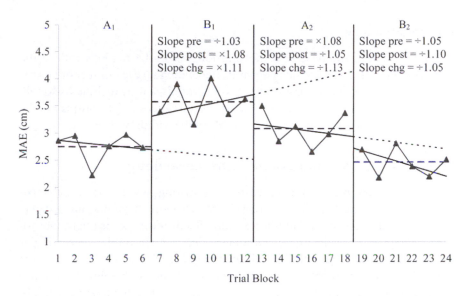

FIGURE 5.8 Split-middle analysis, case number 2. Reprinted with permission from C. Mesagno, D. Marchant and T. Morris (2008) A pre-performance routine to alleviate choking in 'choking-susceptible' athletes, *The Sport Psychologist, 22*, 439–457.

Overall, this study is an example of a well-controlled A–B–A–C design and in particular illustrates how the design allows researchers to explore the effect of interventions and situation (i.e., pressure) manipulations on behaviour whilst ensuring scientific rigour.

A further example is demonstrated by Crouch, Ward and Patrick (1997) who used three variations of the withdrawal design to assess the effects that group instruction, peer dyads and peer-mediated accountability (i.e., teacher-established goals, peer recording of performance, public posting of student performance, and activities that served as public recognition of student achievement) had on the number of trials performed, and the success of the trials, during one-minute trials of volleyball skills. Their sample comprised sixty-seven elementary physical education students across grades four to six. The experimental conditions of the study were as follows: group instruction (A), peer dyads (B) and peer-mediated accountability (C). In grade four, a multi-treatment withdrawal design was used with experimental conditions in the following order: A–B–A–C. This design allowed a direct comparison between each condition. In grade five, the conditions were presented as B–A–C–A, and in grade six the order of the conditions was C–A–C–A. Overall, data indicated that students performed more trials and were generally more successful in the peer-mediated accountability condition than during the peer dyads or group instruction conditions.

Interim summary

The above sections outline some of the common A–B–A–B variations. Indeed, the A–B–A–B design can be extended or varied depending on the number of phases, interventions, ordering of phases and types of reversals that are included. Overall, the variation that is used is dependent on the circumstances and the purpose of the project. The chapter concludes with a critique of the withdrawal design.

Problems and limitations of the withdrawal design

Because the withdrawal design is based upon alternating phases to observe changes in behaviour, the need to illustrate reversal of behaviour is paramount in determining causal inferences about intervention effectiveness. Accordingly, most of the problems associated with the withdrawal design focus on the alternating or reversal of behaviour (Kazdin 1982; Kratochwill et al. 1984). First, it is possible that behaviour (e.g., sport performance) will not return to baseline levels once an intervention has been removed or altered (e.g., Bryan 1987; Kazdin 1982). In such a situation it is likely that the intervention was not responsible for the initial change, and moreover that the change was due to some uncontrolled variable(s). For example, an archer may continue with self-practice of a self-talk routine after instructions to withdraw the technique have been delivered by the practitioner or researcher. Indeed, factors such as history, maturation and illness may occur when an intervention is implemented and remain in effect when the intervention is withdrawn (Kazdin 1982). Overall, it is difficult to evaluate the effects of an intervention in a withdrawal design when behaviour does not revert back to baseline. Second, although the reversal of behaviour to baseline is an important facet of the withdrawal design, it is also an issue of much controversy, as returning behaviour to baseline can make a person 'worse' again and may be considered unethical (Kazdin 1978; Kratochwill et al. 1984). In addition, for some individuals it may not be appropriate for an effective intervention to be removed because the participant may feel uncomfortable as they fear their performance will suffer as a consequence (Bryan 1987; Heyman 1987). Clearly, a paradox exists here for researchers and practitioners. Should we continue to promote human welfare and well-being, or compromise this in pursuit of determining effective interventions? Overall, in clinical settings the consequences of removing an intervention and making a participant worse need to be thoughtfully considered. In situations in which concerns about the ethics of removing an intervention exist, using an alternative design strategy such as the multiple-baseline design (Chapter 6), which does not require removing treatment, may be pertinent.

Evaluation of the design

The withdrawal design, and in particular the A–B–A–B variation, provides researchers and practitioners with a platform to collect clear evidence regarding causal inferences and intervention effectiveness. Typically, this evidence comes from a clear pattern change in behaviour between baseline, issuing of the intervention and then a return to baseline and re-issuing of the intervention. Although the issues of reversing behaviour and removing interventions are problematic, they are important facets of the withdrawal design in allowing for causal inferences about intervention effectiveness to be made. The design variations associated with the withdrawal design are all appropriate for the domains of sport and exercise and selection will very much depend on the needs of the participant and their situational demands. Overall, a strategy for dealing with the ethical dilemma of establishing a lengthy baseline is the B–A–B design. In this design it is possible to move from an immediate treatment condition to a (shortened) baseline. This variation is appropriate for those working in professional sport and exercise settings when establishing a traditional baseline cannot be achieved (e.g., crisis interventions) because of time constraints and pressure from the client, coaches, parents and exercise instructors.

Summary

The withdrawal (including the A–B–A–B variation) design represents a powerful tool for demonstrating intervention effectiveness. However, despite the prevalence of the withdrawal design in mainstream clinical settings, the design has received much less research attention in the areas of sport and exercise. In the withdrawal design the effect of an intervention is usually demonstrated by alternating baseline and intervention phases over time and observing changes in the patterns of behaviour across these phases. Design variations are determined by the order of the baseline and interventions phases, the number of phases and the number of different interventions presented in a design that fit the needs and requirements of the participant and situation. The withdrawal phase is a key characteristic of the design. However, in some cases behaviour does not reverse (causing problems in determining intervention effectiveness) and in others it is undesirable or indeed unethical to withdraw a treatment. When the withdrawal design is considered inappropriate for ethical and logistical reasons there are alternative single-case designs to evaluate intervention effectiveness. We will describe these in the following chapters.

Key points

- The A–B design is a simple single-case design in which data are collected on a target behaviour and then compared with data collected post intervention.
- The withdrawal design is a single-case research design in which baseline phases (A) and treatment phases (B) are alternated. It is also referred to as a reversal or A–B–A design. The design includes variations such as A–B–A–B and B–A–B designs.

- The baseline phase, in which observation of a dependent variable takes place over time, unaffected by the intervention, is a crucial aspect of single-case designs.
- A steady state is when the measured dependent variable displays stability and does not substantially change in an upwards or downwards direction before the presentation of an intervention.
- Behavioural cyclicity includes normal cycles and fluctuations in behaviour prior to intervention as a result of physiological and environmental factors.
- Internal validity is the extent to which changes in the dependent variable can be inferred to be as a consequence of the independent variable (i.e., intervention or treatment).

Guided study

Based upon your reading of Chapter 5, please take some time to respond to the following review questions:

- What is the role of a baseline in single-case research methodology?
- What are the fundamental aspects of a baseline phase?
- What is the major premise behind the withdrawal design?
- What are the strengths and weakness of the withdrawal design for practitioners and researchers?

6

MULTIPLE-BASELINE DESIGNS IN SPORT AND EXERCISE

In this chapter, we will:

- outline the rationale for multiple-baseline designs in sport and exercise;
- outline variations of the multiple-baseline design;
- provide guidance on using the multiple-baseline design in applied sport and exercise contexts.

CASE EXAMPLE

Duncan is a twenty-nine-year-old male professional basketball player who plays as point guard. For the past five years he has moved around from club to club and thus lived in different houses and areas. Over the last six months Duncan has noticed that his overall belief as a basketball player and the belief in his ability to undertake tasks during games (e.g., make assists and simple passes) have substantially decreased, leading to a number of poor performances. In addition, as a result of this apparent loss of confidence and the poor performances, a change in his mood state prior to and after his games has been noted. Typically, this negative affective state is making him feel irritable, angry and frustrated. Duncan has recently been dropped from the team because of his poor performances and therefore feels de-motivated about training and basketball in general and has started to become apprehensive about his future as a professional basketball player. The psychologist working with him has concluded that he is experiencing a lack of self-efficacy (i.e., a belief in one's capabilities to be successful at a given task), which in turn is affecting his mood.

Introduction and basic rationale for the design

In the previous chapter we explained the classic withdrawal research design (A–B–A–B), which has been outlined to be a robust and effective mechanism for evaluating behaviour change in participants in relation to outcome variables (e.g., constructs, performance and behaviour) during applied interventions. Because of the strong reliance on intra-subject replication, the A–B–A–B design allows researchers and practitioners to draw conclusions about participant change, which is one of the main reasons why the design is held in such high regard (see Barlow et al. 2009; Kazdin 1982; Morgan and Morgan 2009). Despite the positive aspects of the withdrawal approach, problems arise when changes in outcome measures (e.g., performance and behaviour) remain permanent and thus are unlikely to return to baseline. There are also ethical concerns about removing a treatment following positive changes (Bryan 1987). In multiple-baseline designs, intervention effects are evaluated using a method quite different from that described for A–B–A–B designs (Kazdin 1982). Typically, effects are demonstrated by introducing the intervention to different baselines (e.g., behaviours, participants, settings, situations and conditions) at different points in time. If changes are observed in each baseline when the intervention is introduced then the effects can be attributed to the intervention rather than variables out of the control of the researcher or practitioner (e.g., weather and pitch conditions, coach, parent or exercise leader instruction). One of the key aspects of this design is that, once the intervention has been presented to alter behaviour, it does not need to be withdrawn and there is no need to return the target behaviour to or near to baseline levels. Overall, the multiple-baseline design avoids the ethical concerns raised in the A–B–A–B design by not withdrawing the intervention when a change in behaviour has been instigated, and so it is one of the most commonly used single-subject designs in the area of sport and exercise (Bryan 1987; Hrycaiko and Martin 1996). This chapter begins with an overview of the design and examples from the sport and exercise literature. Next we consider variations of the multiple-baseline design (i.e., across participants, settings and behaviours, and multiple-probe) and provide further illustrations from the literature. The chapter concludes with an evaluation of the design including its strengths and limitations, and guidance for scientists and practitioners.

In multiple-baseline designs, inferences are typically based on examining target variable(s) across several different baselines or participants, behaviours and/or settings. For example, a coach may be interested in how a positive reflection task in which the athletes focus on three positive aspects of the training session or competition has an impact on motivation across athletes (participants) or changes attendance rates and effort in training and competition (behaviours) or influences effort in training and then competition (settings). Hypothetical data outlined in Figure 6.1 help to demonstrate the major premise of multiple-baseline designs. Baseline data are gathered for each participant or

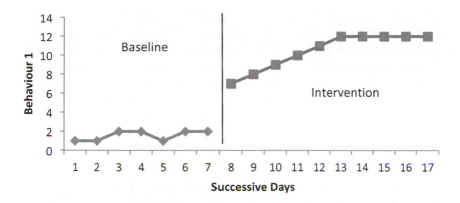

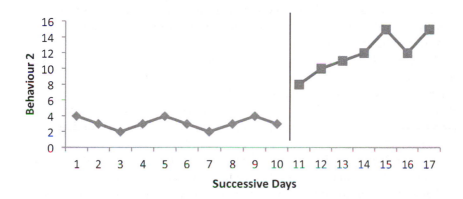

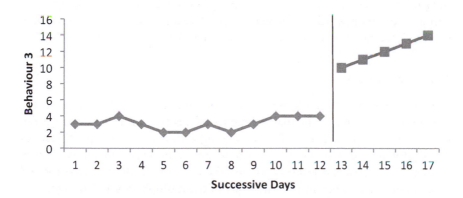

FIGURE 6.1 The multiple-baseline design.

target variable and serve the same purposes common to single-case research (see Chapter 3 for more commentary on this aspect). In other words, data for each baseline describe the current level of the target variable and allow for future performance of this variable to be predicted and inferred. Generally, after the stabilization of the target variable for all baselines, the intervention is applied to the first baseline. Data continue to be gathered for each behaviour, or person, or setting. If the intervention is effective, changes in the target variable (e.g., behaviour) to which the intervention was applied are observed. Participants, behaviours or settings yet to receive the intervention at this stage should remain consistent in their baseline target variable. Data at this stage are not clear and conclusive about intervention effectiveness and will only be considered so when observed changes noted for behaviour or participant 1 are replicated across the remaining baselines following introduction of the intervention. Therefore, once performance stabilizes across all target variables the intervention is applied to the second baseline (participant). Thus at this point both the first and second baselines are receiving the intervention to bring about changes in the target variable, and data continue to be obtained for all target variables. Finally, the intervention is applied to the third participant while data continue to be gathered on all three.

The multiple-baseline design demonstrates the effect of an intervention by illustrating that changes in target variables take place when *and only when* an intervention is applied. For example, in Figure 6.1 the pattern of data implies that whenever, and to whomever, the intervention is applied, changes in the target variable are observed, thereby ruling out the possible confounding effect of extraneous variables.

As with A–B–A–B designs, multiple-baseline designs are based on testing predictions. For example, each time the intervention is applied, the researcher makes a prediction about how an intervention may help to bring about a change from baseline to post-intervention data. Therefore, each baseline is a mini-experiment of sorts, with the aim of providing researchers and practitioners with a model with which to facilitate their drawing of conclusions regarding intervention efficacy and effectiveness (Seligman 1995).

Design variations

The basic rationale for the multiple-baseline design has been outlined in the previous section. One of the major benefits of this type of design is that it can be varied to reflect the needs of what is being assessed. For example, baselines can be created for different individuals or groups or different situations, settings or times. The following sections provide the reader with the rationale for and guidance on the more common variations of the multiple-baseline design.

Multiple-baseline across-participants design

In this variation of the design, baseline data are gathered for a particular target variable performed by two or more individuals. Thus, the multiple baselines refer to the number of persons whose target variables are being observed.

Typically, the researcher or practitioner begins by collecting observations (data) of the same baseline target variables (e.g., confidence, mood, inappropriate behaviour, performance) for each person. After the variable has reached a stable rate (in the baseline phase), the intervention is applied to one participant, while baseline conditions are continued for the other(s). In essence, the variable of the person exposed to the intervention is proposed to change, while for the other participants the variable is proposed to continue at the baseline levels. When the target variable stabilizes for all individuals, the intervention is extended to another person. This process is repeated until all of the individuals for whom baseline data were collected receive the intervention. The effect of the intervention is demonstrated when a change in each person's target variable is obtained at the point when the intervention is introduced and not before (Barlow and Hersen 1984; Kazdin 1982; Martin and Pear 2003).

You may recall Duncan from our case study earlier in the chapter – he was a professional basketball player suffering with debilitating self-efficacy (i.e., a lack of belief in his ability to be successful as a basketball player) and negative affect. The psychologist working with Duncan decided to use an imagery intervention programme to enhance his self-efficacy. To ensure that any increase in Duncan's self-efficacy was a consequence of the imagery intervention, and not some other uncontrolled variable, the psychologist decided to evaluate the programme using a multiple-baseline design. To do this, the psychologist provided the intervention at different times for Duncan and two other clients, Tommy and Roger, who were also experiencing debilitating self-efficacy. Thus the study began with the collection of baseline data from all three clients, as illustrated in Figure 6.2.

You will notice from Figure 6.2 that the baseline phases are unequal and the intervention is delivered to the clients at different times. This staggered or unequal baseline is what gives the design its alternative name of a *staggered* baseline design. Each client receives the intervention once and only one phase change from baseline to treatment occurs during the study for each client.

Exclusive to the multiple-baseline design is the fact that there is no return to baseline after treatment, unlike the A–B–A–B withdrawal design, and that participants are allowed to act as their own controls, where appropriate. Overall, the design represents a simple A–B design (see Chapter 5), but is nevertheless replicated to establish the reliability of the intervention effect. Accordingly, the internal validity of this design is ensured by the multiple replications of the intervention delivered across clients, settings or behaviour (Kazdin 2003). Moreover, each transition from baseline to treatment is an opportunity for the researcher to observe treatment effects and draw conclusions about the intervention. Indeed, making this transition at different times allows the researcher to rule out alternative explanations for any target variable change post treatment. In addition, if this change were instigated at the same time for all three clients, changes in the target behaviour would prove difficult to interpret as it is possible that some extraneous variable (e.g., coach instruction or encouragement, historical event) could have coincided with the start of the intervention and

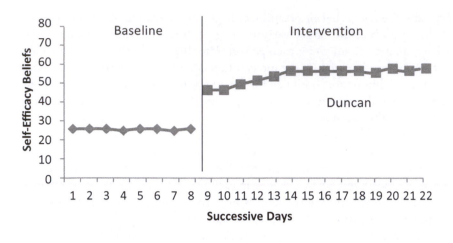

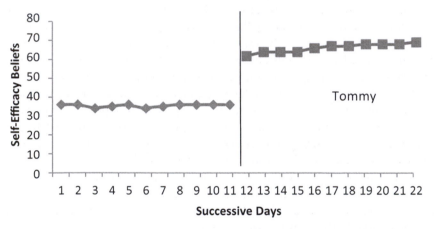

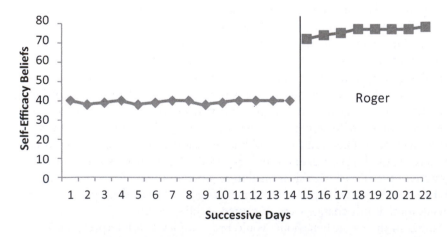

FIGURE 6.2 The multiple-baseline across-participants design.

had a comparable influence on all three clients' target variable. Although the likelihood of this occurring is low, it could happen, and so it is important to rule it out.

The major strength of the across-participants variation of the design is that if each participant's target variable remains stable during baseline, and changes only when the intervention is presented, then one can be quite sure that a treatment effect has occurred and that any change is not due to the influence of some uncontrolled variable. In essence, the multiple-baseline design, by allowing for several baseline-to-treatment phase changes at different points in time, is a powerful single-subject alternative to the withdrawal design (Kinugasa et al. 2004).

When looking to adopt the across-participants design variation a stable baseline is as important as in any other single-case design. For example, variability in the baseline data or a noticeable trend in the direction of the intended outcome can make it difficult to determine intervention effectiveness. On occasions, particularly when working with athletes from the same team, group or organization, it is possible that increases may be seen in other participants once they begin to interact (e.g., talking to one another about the sport psychology advice they have been provided with). Therefore, one should pay particular attention to minimizing this effect during the design (Morgan and Morgan 2009).

In Figure 6.2 you will notice that each measure of the target variable during baseline occurs at the same time (e.g., on successive days) for each participant before the intervention is presented. However, it is not always the case in practice that participants are being monitored and their target variables recorded and measured at precisely the same time (e.g., on the same successive days as each other). Indeed, researchers (Kazdin 1982; Morgan and Morgan 2009) have made the distinction between *concurrent* multiple-baseline designs (in which simultaneous measurement occurs for all participants) and *non-concurrent* multiple-baseline designs (when data collection does not occur simultaneously). In the latter case, participants do not begin the baseline at exactly the same time. Thus, it is quite possible that data for both the baseline and treatment phases may be collected for one participant before the baseline data are collected for the others. For example, data may be collected on one netball player during the first five weeks of the season before the psychologist moves on to work with another player using an identical intervention. Concurrent measurement controls better for threats to internal validity. However, researchers publishing multiple-baseline studies may fail to clarify if the data are concurrent or non-concurrent, making it difficult to infer the timing of their data collection (Carr 2005). This is also the case in the sport and exercise literature (Lindsay, Maynard and Thomas 2005). Glancing further at Figure 6.2 it is obvious how readers often assume that data have been collected at the same points in time. Indeed, the drawing of this conclusion is a common pitfall for researchers plotting data onto graphs. The reality is that, for many practitioners working in applied sport and exercise contexts, they will seldom work with clients sharing the same problems at exactly the same time. Accordingly, the use of non-concurrent multiple-baseline designs has been supported based on the notion that they reflect the real essence of carrying out interventions in the real world (e.g., Carr 2005; Harvey, May and Kennedy 2004; Lindsay et al. 2005).

The multiple-baseline across-participants design is especially useful for situations in which a particular target variable or set of target variables in need of change is constant among different people. For example, it may be that a coach is trying to improve the frequency of positive encouragement amongst his defensive players in a netball team, or a sport psychologist may wish to enhance the collective efficacy (i.e., beliefs that a group hold about being able to successfully accomplish specific tasks) of an Olympic four-man bobsleigh team. In this type of design, no reversal or experimental conditions are required to demonstrate the effects of the intervention. The following section provides a synopsis of research using across-participants variations in sport and exercise.

Multiple-baseline across-participants designs in sport and exercise: illustrations

The multiple-baseline across-participants design (Barlow and Hersen 1984; Martin and Pear 2003) has been suggested to be one of the most pertinent methods for use in applied sport psychology research given that practitioners are often required to work with participants from the same team, thereby sharing similar performance-related issues (see Bryan 1987; Hrycaiko and Martin 1996). As such, the design remains one of the most common methods to ascertain intervention efficacy and effectiveness within the sport psychology literature (e.g., Callow, Hardy and Hall 2001; Callow and Waters 2005; Calmels, Berthoumieux and d'Arripe-Longueville 2004; Freeman et al. 2009; Galvan and Ward 1998; Hanton and Jones 1999; Mellalieu et al. 2009; Pates, Oliver and Maynard 2001; Thelwell and Greenlees 2001). To illustrate, Galvan and Ward (1998) used a multiple-baseline design across five players to assess the effectiveness of a public posting intervention in reducing inappropriate on-court behaviours (e.g., verbal abuse by a player during a match). The study involved observing players concurrently (collecting data) throughout the season during weekly challenge matches. A staggered baseline was used with two participants receiving the intervention after six baseline measures, another two participants after ten baseline measures and one participant after fourteen baseline measures. The first intervention phase involved initial feedback on inappropriate behaviours and an explanation of the intervention procedures and goal-setting. In the second phase, the number of inappropriate behaviours for each player was posted. Results indicated that the intervention was effective in immediately reducing the number of inappropriate on-court behaviours for all players (see Figure 6.3).

Hanton and Jones (1999) examined the effects of a multi-modal intervention on swimmers debilitated by anxiety. A staggered single-subject multiple-baseline across-participants design was used for four swimmers over ten competitive

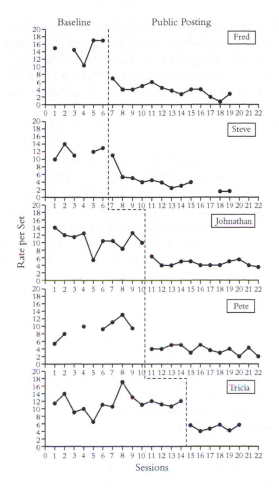

FIGURE 6.3 Number of inappropriate behaviours per set for each player during baseline and intervention. Adapted with permission from Z. J. Galvan and P. Ward (1998) Effects of public posting on inappropriate on-court behaviors by collegiate tennis players. *The Sport Psychologist, 12*, 419–426.

races. Interestingly, one participant acted as a control, even though a multiple-baseline design negates the need for this (Kazdin 2003), whilst the others received the intervention comprising goal-setting, imagery and self-talk after three, four and five baseline measures (pre-race data) respectively. Data indicated meaningful changes in anxiety perception with all three experimental participants reporting facilitative interpretations. Performance improvements were also evident for these swimmers. A five-month follow-up data collection phase of pre-race thoughts before two races per participant indicated anxiety perceptions were still facilitative. The follow-up used is an important aspect of this study as it provides information about the long-term benefits of applied interventions (Gardner and Moore 2006).

Haddad and Tremayne (2009) investigated the effectiveness of a centring concentration technique involving breath control on the free-throw shooting percentage of young athletes aged ten to eleven years. A convenience sample was used involving young representative basketball players (juniors who were tri-alled, selected and identified as the most talented basketball players in their age group). The sample consisted of two girls and three boys (mean = 10 years and 7 months, standard deviation = 6 months) from a basketball stadium located in Sydney, Australia. The participants trained at least twice a week and played representative games against other metropolitan associations at the weekends. A multiple-baseline across-participants design was used. During the baseline period participants were monitored until they were deemed ready for the intervention, which occurred at different times for each participant. Hence, each participant needed to have established a stable baseline (i.e., a consistent free-throw shooting percentage, data points within a 5–10 per cent range) or their data points needed to have displayed a trend that was headed in the opposite direction to that anticipated after the intervention (Hrycaiko and Martin 1996). The baseline period for all participants ranged from two to three weeks with two shooting sessions per week. Therefore, baseline lengths ranged from four to six data points. The intervention period, which involved a twenty-minute session on the centring breath, followed the baseline period. The post-intervention phase was conducted over a four-week period (i.e., eight shooting sessions). Data revealed that the centring breath was a useful tool for improving all participants' performance to varying degrees. To illustrate, Figure 6.4 reveals an immediate and maintained shooting percentage performance increase following the intervention for participant 3.

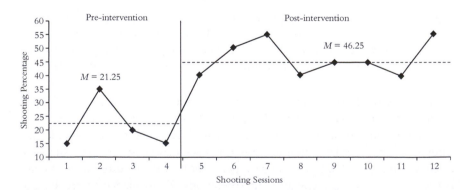

FIGURE 6.4 Participant 3's free-throw shooting percentage for shooting sessions during the pre- and post-intervention phases. Adapted with permission from K. Haddad and P. Tremayne (2009) The effects of centering on the free-throw shooting performance of young athletes. *The Sport Psychologist,* *23,* 118–136.

Interim summary

In summary, multiple-baseline across-participants designs involve replication of an A–B phase change delivered in a staggered fashion over time across two or more participants. Each replication of the intervention allows inferences to be made regarding the internal validity of the intervention because the staggered baseline eliminates alternative explanations for behaviour change (Kazdin 1982). Moreover, the across-participants variation increases the external validity of an intervention because of inter-subject replications. The across-participants design has been a common design in the sport and exercise literature because it lends itself well to the issues and demands that practitioners face (Kinugasa et al. 2004).

Multiple-baseline across-settings/situations design

When working or researching individuals in sport and exercise settings, there is often a need to evaluate intervention effectiveness for a client or a client group across different situations (e.g., training, home and away performance, exercising with a personal trainer, exercising with a group, exercising alone at home). In such situations we are interested in intra-subject replication. This is achieved by way of a multiple-baseline across-settings/situations design. In this design, interventions are staggered for the individual or group across different settings and/or environments that they typically encounter (e.g., two or three different environments or settings). The same target variable is measured in each of the identified settings and/or situations. To illustrate, a professional basketball team have reported a high frequency of inappropriate on-court behaviours during tournaments and practice matches in training. The sport psychologist recommends using public posting (e.g., publishing a record of players' behaviours during matches), revealing the frequency of inappropriate behaviours by the players as recorded by their coach. In this situation the intervention is implemented in a staggered fashion across the two different environments: (1) tournaments and (2) non-tournaments (including practice matches and training). Figure 6.5 illustrates the collection of baseline data regarding the frequency of inappropriate on-court behaviours in both tournaments and practice matches in training. The prevalence of inappropriate on-court behaviours is evidently reduced following the presentation of the intervention in a staggered manner.

As in other multiple-baseline designs, several phase changes from baseline to treatment are key in this variation to establishing intervention effectiveness. Ideally, practitioners and clients want to see changes in target variables in all environments (e.g., practice and competition), otherwise the intervention may be considered unsuccessful. The major benefit of the multiple-baseline across-settings design is that it is useful in determining the effects of interventions when the needs of a client or group cross over many situations. Moreover, multiple-baseline designs derive strength from multiple A–B (baseline to treatment)

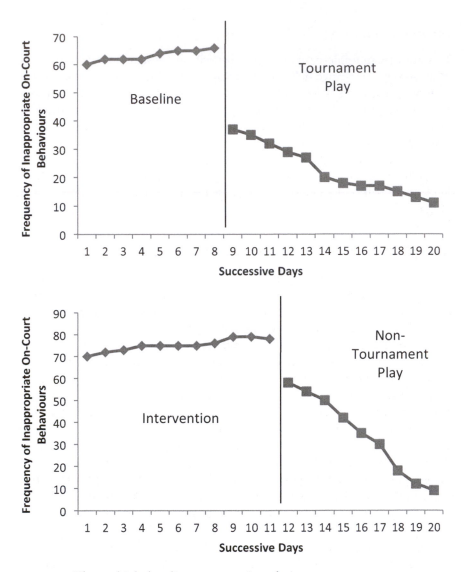

FIGURE 6.5 The multiple-baseline across-settings design.

phase changes staggered over time. In essence, the more replications provided in a single study, the more confident the researcher or practitioner can be about the effects of the intervention. To illustrate, Kazdin (1994) recommends two or three separate baseline phases as a minimum to allow for one or two replications of the original effect, leading to the drawing of stronger conclusions. Of course, the number of replications will very much depend on the needs of the client group, the opportunities available to the researchers and the constraints of working in applied practice (e.g., feasibility of data collection). Whilst this section has outlined the rationale behind the across-settings variation, the following section outlines specific research adopting this approach in sport and exercise settings.

Multiple-baseline across-settings/situations designs in sport and exercise: illustrations

Despite the obvious appeal of the across-settings variation in sport and exercise, very little research has been published adopting this approach with participants in sport and exercise settings. One explanation is that it is very difficult to keep the effect of the intervention constrained to one setting. In the example provided earlier (Figure 6.5) of an intervention with a basketball team to reduce inappropriate on-court behaviours it is difficult to imagine that behaving more appropriately in practice will not, at least partially, transfer to competition. A second explanation is that there has been inadequate training in the use of single-case research methods in undergraduate and postgraduate psychology and sport science courses.

In a study by Allen (1998) an enhanced simplified habit-reversal (SHR) procedure (including awareness training, teaching a competing response and arranging supporting contingencies that are likely to strengthen the use of the competing response; Miltenberger, Fuqua and McKinley 1985; Woods, Miltenberger and Lumley 1996) was used with a fourteen-year-old boy. The boy presented with a long history of disruptive, angry outbursts during tennis matches (i.e., loud verbal self-deprecation, smacking his tennis racket on the court, slapping his hat against his legs, and waving his arms in the air in response to missed shots, lost points or situations in which he may have won the point but felt he made a poor decision or used poor technique). Baseline data were collected independently by the player and his parents on numbers of outbursts during four non-tournament and six tournament matches to assess the player's awareness and rate. Using a staggered multiple-baseline across-settings design (i.e., non-tournament and tournament), SHR procedures were delivered along with continual data collection from non-tournament and tournament settings. Because of modest results following the SHR, an enhanced SHR procedure (e.g., response–cost procedure in which failure to immediately terminate outbursts led to the participant's withdrawal from tennis practice) was incorporated. Overall, results revealed elimination of disruptive outbursts in both settings, which was further supported by twelve-month follow-up data collected by the player's parents. Figure 6.6 details an obvious trend in which there is a reduction in outbursts from baseline to treatment phases.

This study is a useful example of the across-settings design and, like the Hanton and Jones (1999) study described earlier in the chapter, also highlights the importance of monitoring long-term intervention effects (Martin, Vause and Schwartzman 2005).

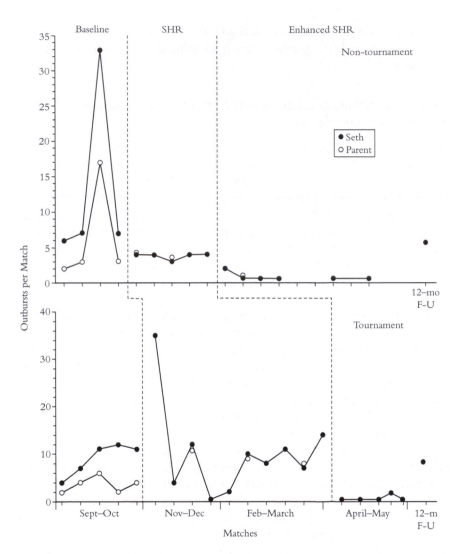

FIGURE 6.6 Outbursts per match reported by Seth and his parents across non-tournament and tournament matches, during baseline and both the SHR and the enhanced SHR procedures. Adapted with permission from K. Allen (1998) Variable effects of a behavioral treatment package on the performance of inline roller speed skaters. *Journal of Applied Behavior Analysis, 35*, 489–492.

Interim summary

The across-settings variation is an important aspect of multiple-baseline designs because intervention effectiveness is determined through replication across a number of settings as opposed to individuals. Such a design may therefore be well suited to interventions whose objective is to bring about changes in target variables in one or more relevant sport and exercise environments. On this basis researchers and practitioners should adopt this design more often in their applied work, so adding to the extant sport and exercise literature regarding across-settings approaches (Zaichkowsky 1980).

Multiple-baseline across-behaviours designs

One of the major benefits of multiple-baseline designs is that to assess an intervention one does not require a large sample size – only several opportunities to replicate the intervention. Therefore, the logic of the multiple-baseline across-behaviours design is to collect different responses and/or different facets of an individual's behavioural locker. Figure 6.7 highlights an across-behaviours design for a newly qualified soccer coach delivering coaching sessions to an under-14 team.

As you can imagine, the coach wished to improve his coaching instruction during sessions. The coach's mentor suggested an intervention comprising education on effective communication and self-reflection. Therefore, the frequency of positive encouragement, punishment and demonstrations in each coaching session was monitored and three baselines were created. As depicted in Figure 6.7, there was very little positive encouragement and few demonstrations, whereas punishment was a more common occurrence. The mentor implemented the first intervention phase for the behaviour of positive encouragement whilst the other two behaviours continued in baseline. After several training sessions the intervention was then applied to the second behaviour (punishment). Finally, the intervention was applied several training sessions later to the last behaviour (demonstrations).

In this type of design, replication of the intervention occurs for the same participant or clients but across different target variables or dimensions of target variables (e.g., passing and shooting, stretching and cooling down). Accordingly, each targeted variable must be objectively defined and the dimensions clearly designated to ensure measurement rigour. Moreover, in this design (as with other multiple-baseline designs) it is likely that there will be some carry-over of the intervention from one variable (i.e., behaviour) to another. For example, baseline data for one variable (e.g., concentration) may be seen to be increasing near the end of the baseline period. Because this trend corresponds to the intervention phase for the first variable (e.g., anxiety) this increase is often referred to as 'behavioural covariation'. Behavioural covariation is when changes in non-targeted variables (e.g., behaviour) occur as a consequence of them being similar to those targeted by the intervention (Sprague and Horner 1992).

When dealing with a number of different dimensions of a target variable (e.g., behaviour) there is a possibility that they will interact with or influence one another. This interaction (known as the 'behavioural cusp'; Rosales-Ruiz and Baer 1997) causes difficulty in drawing conclusions about intervention effectiveness, although it can be clinically useful, particularly if positive changes

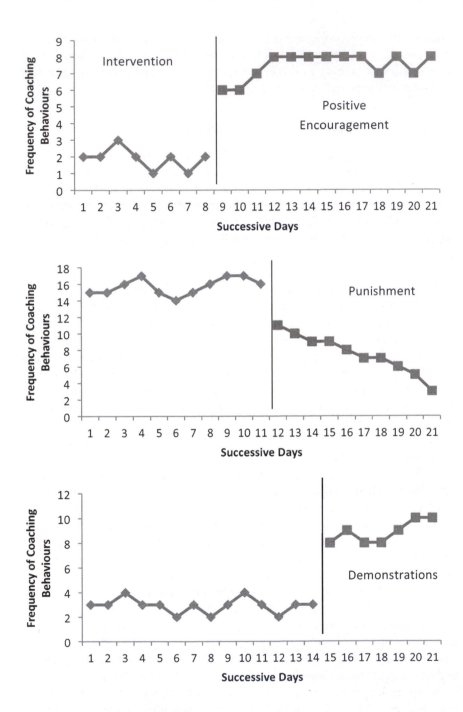

FIGURE 6.7 The multiple-baseline across-behaviours design.

in target variables are observed. In relation to the coaching example in Figure 6.7, it is possible that punishment occurs less frequently and demonstrations more frequently during the first intervention because the education received relative to positive encouragement promotes a broader reflection on effective communication by the coach. Such an occurrence, although problematic for the researcher, is potentially useful for a practitioner. To explain, an intervention that brings about changes in not only the specified behaviour but also other related behaviours is regarded positively. Typically, behavioural cusps are desirable (particularly for practitioners) and are an unplanned by-product of an intervention, although they make the drawing of cause and effect conclusions difficult. Practitioners should consider the potential for behavioural cusps when developing intervention programmes (Morgan and Morgan 2009). The above section has outlined the main considerations for a multiple-baseline across-behaviours variation. The following section provides examples of how this design has been used within sport and exercise settings.

Multiple-baseline across-behaviours designs in sport and exercise: illustrations

Similar to multiple-baseline designs across settings, examples of the multiple-baseline design across behaviours are scant in the sport and exercise literature despite the obvious appeal of providing researchers and practitioners with a framework to assess intervention effectiveness across two or more target variables. To illustrate, McKenzie and Rushall (1974) used an across-behaviours variation in experiment one of a two-experiment study on a group of thirty-two swimmers whose attendance at training was described by their coaches as being poor and irregular. Treatment consisting of self-recording attendance on a publicly posted attendance board was made contingent first on simply showing up and swimming (reduce absence), then on being on time and swimming (reduce tardiness), and finally on showing up on time, swimming and staying for the entire practice (reduce instances of leaving early). Data revealed that the frequencies of absenteeism, late arrival and early departure were reduced following the self-recorded public posting intervention. Moreover, post-checks conducted three weeks after the intervention period indicated that the attendance board remained effective in controlling the problems of attendance. Figure 6.8 details the reduction in behaviours following the intervention.

Rushall and Smith (1979) used an across-behaviours variation to monitor the effects of a self-recording intervention in a competitive swimming training situation to change the repertoire, quality and quantity of several behaviour categories in a coach. Self-recording techniques were used for rewarding, providing feedback and providing feedback after first rewarding a swimmer. The repertoire of behaviours in these categories was increased through the provision of discriminative stimuli on self-recording sheets. Fading schedules (i.e., a method for providing reinforcement) were successfully used to reduce the

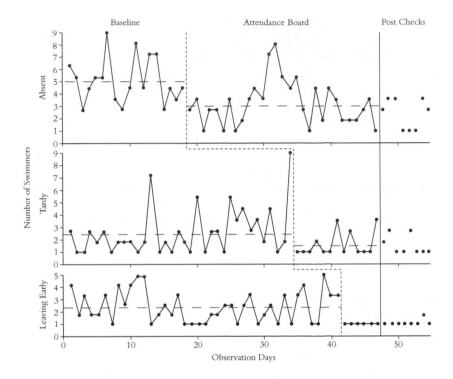

FIGURE 6.8 The number of swimmers who were absent, arrived late and left early during baseline and experimental conditions. Adapted with permission from T. L. McKenzie and B. S. Rushall (1974) Effects of self-recording on attendance and performance in a competitive swimming training environment. *Journal of Applied Behavior Analysis*, 7, 199–206.

coach's reliance on the prompt sheets. Rates of occurrence of the target behaviours served as a reinforcing procedure for increasing the emission frequencies. A learning of schedule reinforcement produced a persistent change in the scope and quantity of the outcome behaviours. Pre- and post-experimental behaviour analyses of the coach observation schedule indicated that the affected changes also produced concomitant changes in other behavioural categories (i.e., managerial activities, feedback, directing, explaining and informing, rewarding).

Finally, Swain and Jones (1995) used an across-behaviours variation to examine the effects of a goal-setting intervention programme on selected components of basketball performance (i.e., offensive rebounds, defensive rebounds, steals, turnovers, assists, shot percentage from the field, shot percentage from the foul line, fouls) over the course of a competitive season. At a mid-season break, four elite college basketball players selected one aspect of their play that they felt would benefit from improvement. A goal-setting intervention was designed based on a goal-attainment scaling procedure (Smith 1988) in which participants generated numerical targets for their chosen components. These components were then measured for eight games in the post-intervention phase. Three of the four participants showed consistent improvements in their targeted behaviours. In addition, social validation data (Kazdin 1982) indicated that three of the four participants had been highly committed to improvement on their target, that the goal-setting procedure had been useful and acceptable, and that the intervention had had a substantial effect on the participants' performance components.

The collection of social validation data from coaches, athletes, parents and exercisers in the form of questionnaires or interviews is considered an important aspect of single-case methods (Kazdin 1982) and is explained in more detail in Chapter 4. In short, social validation allows for the measurement of perceptions of intervention effectiveness, costliness and likelihood of intervention implementation in the future. In the case of multiple-baseline designs, social validation can assist researchers and practitioners in understanding the formulation and effects of behavioural cusps and covariation. The prevalence of social validation procedures being reported in the sport and exercise literature has recently increased (e.g., Barker, Jones and Greenlees 2010; Hanton and Jones 1999) because researchers now recognize the importance of this information in determining intervention efficacy as well as effectiveness (Seligman 1995).

Interim summary

The across-behaviours variation permits the replication of an A–B phase change within the same participant or participant group. The behaviours variation is appropriate for sport and exercise because interventions can be assessed across more than one targeted variable. In this type of design, behavioural covariation is likely to occur because intervening with one participant or behaviour may transfer over to non-targeted participants or behaviours. Although covariation effects can be problematic in drawing cause and effect inferences regarding interventions, they along with behavioural cusps represent an important by-product that can bring about meaningful clinical effects for participants.

Multiple-probe designs

Despite the user-friendly nature of the multiple-baseline design in determining intervention effectiveness, it often needs to be adapted to reflect the real-world contingencies of working with sport and exercise clients and/or client groups. However, adapting the design to meet applied demands may compromise scientific measurement. To illustrate, the multiple-baseline design involves the use of separate baselines, staggering of an intervention and baselines becoming progressively longer. Such aspects make this design problematic in applied settings as it is not always feasible to obtain data over lengthy baseline phases, particularly if participants see others in a team, or training group, receiving an intervention that may be beneficial. Moreover, a participant in a sport and exercise setting may require a 'crisis' intervention such that a practitioner cannot dwell on scientific rigour by collating standard baselines because it is unethical to ask the participant for a repeated measurement in such circumstances.

A complication that may make the collection of a conventional baseline futile is the fact that the targeted variable (e.g., a behaviour) may not exist in a participant's repertoire (Barlow et al. 2009). For example, prior to education regarding pre-performance routines, the frequency of their use by a group of young golfers may be zero. Thus the repeated measurement of this baseline behaviour is perhaps pointless and unethical in this context because the baseline behaviour has not yet been acquired by the golfers. Under such circumstances, researchers and practitioners are encouraged to use a multiple-probe design (Horner and Baer 1978). In essence, in this design baseline assessment of the target variable entails quick probes, rather than repeated or continuous measurement. This variation represents an important addition for the sport and exercise community because it is more flexible to the demands of applied consultancy in comparison with other multiple-baseline variations. A probe is characterized as a single discrete measurement of a target variable (e.g., exercise enjoyment), which is often random with no predetermined time (e.g., non-consecutive exercise sessions). The essence of a probe is to establish the natural rate of the target variable (through observation, self-report measures and/or interview) before the intervention, and it is therefore less intrusive than the more traditional multiple-baseline design (Morgan and Morgan 2009). For example, two, three or four simple probes may serve to evaluate the prevalence of pre-performance routines at baseline. Because of this short baseline, typically interventions are delivered with less delay than in other variations. This design is particularly useful if the target behaviour does not occur, or it is stable and does not fluctuate (e.g., a regular exerciser who has attended the gym twice a week for the last six months). In a multiple-probe design, change is determined by comparing data obtained during treatment to that obtained from the pre-intervention probes. In addition, probes are also a useful and non-invasive mechanism for assessing the long-term maintenance effects of an intervention.

Because of the obvious ease with which the multiple-probe design can be used to cater for the specific demands of individuals and groups, this approach has commonly been used by applied scientists (see Barlow et al. 2009; Morgan and Morgan 2009). However, one applied area that has seen little use of the multiple-probe design is the domain of sport and exercise. Indeed, it seems to date that no applied research using this approach has been published.

Interim summary

The multiple-probe design is an adaptation of the multiple-baseline design and involves discrete measurement of targeted variables as opposed to the repeated measures seen in other variations. This approach is commonly used in applied settings where it is not always possible to collect data from a prolonged baseline. Probes are used to assess baseline levels of target variables (e.g., behaviours) that are not known to exist, along with assessing long-term changes and maintenance in target variables following an intervention.

Problems and limitations of the multiple-baseline design

The multiple-baseline design has a series of limitations with regard to determining intervention effectiveness (see Barlow et al. 2009; Kazdin 1982). First, problems can arise from the interdependence of the baselines. To illustrate, for an intervention to be deemed effective, one needs to be sure that changes in each baseline (behaviour, person or situation) occur only when the intervention has been applied and not beforehand. It is common for baselines to be 'interdependent' – in other words, a change in one of the baselines carries over to the others before formal intervention, thereby making it difficult to draw conclusions about treatment effectiveness. This behavioural covariation is particularly likely to arise in the across-behaviours and across-individuals variations because a change in one behaviour (i.e., target variable) or in one individual can influence behaviours and individuals yet to receive the intervention. Second, an intervention may produce inconsistent effects on behaviours, individuals or situations. For example, some behaviours may be altered when the intervention is applied, whereas others are not. Thus in this situation it is likely that some extraneous variable accounted for the change rather than the intervention, calling into question the internal validity of the design or suggesting that the effectiveness of the intervention is the not the same across all participants. In addition, such an inconsistency gives an insight into the overall generality and strength of the intervention (Kazdin 1982). Finally, multiple baselines require the use of prolonged baselines during which the intervention is withheld from each baseline (behaviour, person or situation). Ethically this may be difficult if a participant who would benefit from an intervention has to wait several days or weeks until a stable baseline has been attained. Methodologically, the use of a prolonged baseline may also facilitate changes in target variables before the intervention is applied. To illustrate, participants may develop alternative strategies during a long baseline as a consequence of observation (e.g., the modelling effects of watching teammates perform successfully may facilitate self-efficacy beliefs) and problem solving (e.g., communicating with coaches may provide an athlete with a new training drill). In addition, changes in target variables may be an artefact of repeated testing in which participants become familiar with measures and advocate socially desirable responses.

Evaluation of the design

Notwithstanding the limitations noted, overall the multiple-baseline design has many advantages for researchers and practitioners in sport and exercise contexts (Kazdin 1982; Kinugasa et al. 2004). First, the design (and its related variations) does not depend on the withdrawal of an intervention to determine effectiveness.

Second, it is particularly suited to practical settings because it permits an intervention to be applied to one target variable (person or situation) at a time before it is transferred to other variables. This gradual application of the intervention across different variables is a practical benefit. Finally, the application of an intervention to one variable at a time allows for a test of intervention effectiveness. Assessing the intervention with one target variable or person makes it possible to examine the effects and/or procedure so as to refine the intervention before applying it to the remaining behaviours and individuals.

Summary

The purpose of this chapter was to provide information and guidance on the basic rationale behind the multiple-baseline design and variations of the design and to indicate how best to apply the multiple-baseline design to sport and exercise contexts. The multiple-baseline design represents one of the key methods for determining intervention effectiveness in applied research. The effects of an intervention are typically demonstrated by applying the intervention to different baselines at different points in time. An effect is highlighted when the outcome measures change when, and only when, an intervention is applied. A number of variations to the basic design exist and these have been created to cater for the gathering of multiple baselines across individuals, settings or behaviours. Typically, the designs require a minimum of two baselines to evaluate intervention effectiveness. The strength of this effectiveness is commonly determined by the number of participants, behaviours and/or settings to which the intervention is applied to and is effective for, the stability of each of the baselines, and the magnitude and speed of the changes following the intervention. The main problems of using multiple-baseline designs for applied research focus on the interdependence of baselines, the inconsistent effect of interventions and the collecting of prolonged baselines. The multiple-baseline design remains one of the most common single-case designs within applied research because it does not require reversal to determine change and thus is typically participant friendly.

The prevalence of multiple-baseline designs in the sport and exercise literature to date is scant in comparison with more traditional nomothetic methods (see Hrycaiko and Martin 1996). This lack of use is surprising given the suitability of the multiple baseline to sport and exercise settings, behaviour and participants. Future research could further embrace the multiple-baseline design for determining intervention effectiveness along with the across-settings, across-behaviours and multiple-probe variations. The following chapter looks at another alternative single-case method, the changing-criterion design.

Key points

- The multiple-baseline design is a single-case design incorporating an A–B phase change across subjects, behaviours and/or settings.

- The multiple-baseline across-participants design is a variation incorporating A–B changes in a staggered approach across one or more participants or clients.
- The concurrent multiple-baseline design is when all baseline measures are collected simultaneously.
- The non-concurrent multiple-baseline design is when separate baseline data are not collected simultaneously.
- The multiple-baseline across-settings design is a variation using several A–B phase changes in a staggered fashion across two or more separate settings and/or situations.
- The multiple-baseline across-behaviours design is a variation using several A–B phase changes in a staggered fashion across two or more distinct target behaviours.
- Behavioural covariation is when changes in non-targeted variables occur as a consequence of them being similar to those targeted by the intervention.
- Behavioural cusps relate to the possibility that changes in targeted variables may interact or influence one another as a consequence of intervention.
- Social validation is information collected from the participant, or the participant's family, coaches, teammates, exercisers, that helps to demonstrate and supplement quantitative data regarding intervention effectiveness and efficacy.
- The multiple-probe design is a variation of the multiple-baseline design in which brief 'probes' are taken at baseline and during intervention. It can be used in situations in which the collection of prolonged baselines and repeated measures is unethical and/or does not fit with the needs of the client or the situation.

Guided study

Based upon your reading of Chapter 6 please take some time to respond to the following review questions:

- What is the major assumption underlying the multiple-baseline design?
- How does the multiple-baseline design differ from the A–B–A–B withdrawal design?
- Describe what is meant by 'behavioural covariation'? What are the issues surrounding behavioural covariation in multiple-baseline designs?
- Describe what is meant by 'behavioural cusps'? What are the issues surrounding behavioural cusps in multiple-baseline designs?
- Explain the issues surrounding the use of a probe design in sport and exercise settings.

7

THE CHANGING-CRITERION DESIGN IN SPORT AND EXERCISE

In this chapter, we will:

* outline the rationale for the use of changing-criterion designs in sport and exercise;
* outline variations of the changing-criterion design;
* provide guidance on using the changing-criterion design in applied sport and exercise contexts.

CASE EXAMPLE

Bill is a fifty-six-year-old man who is overweight and suffering with a heart condition. He has previously undertaken very little exercise because of work and family commitments, and a lack of motivation. Bill's general practitioner (GP) recommends that he reduce his body weight to alleviate some of the suffering from his heart condition. He also recommends that Bill should take up regular, structured exercise. Accordingly, Bill is referred to a GP exercise referral scheme at a local health club. Upon Bill's first visit to the club he meets with an exercise psychologist who consults him about his motives, anxieties and barriers to exercise. Based on Bill's responses, the exercise psychologist suggests that he should undertake a regular jogging routine on one of the club's treadmills five times a week with the ultimate aim being to jog continuously for sixty minutes. To help Bill achieve this sixty-minute goal, the exercise psychologist develops an exercise plan intervention. This intervention is focused on increasing the length of time spent jogging by five minutes every time Bill's current behaviour has been maintained for five consecutive jogs.

Introduction and basic rationale for the design

The chapter begins with an overview of the changing-criterion design and examples from the sport and exercise literature. Next we consider variations of the changing-criterion design (e.g., range-bound and distributed-critierion designs) and provide further illustrations from the literature. The chapter concludes with an evaluation of the design including its strengths and limitations, and guidance for scientists and practitioners.

The changing-criterion design is an extension of the withdrawal design (e.g., A–B–A–B; see Chapter 5) in which the intervention effect is demonstrated by showing that target variables change gradually over the course of the intervention phase. A criterion is set that represents a target (goal) for the participant to meet. This criterion (or goal) will change throughout the course of the study. It is anticipated that the variable improves in increments to match the criterion that is specified as part of the intervention (Kazdin 1982). Normally, rewards or incentives are provided to facilitate the attainment of a designated criterion. For example, rest periods (e.g., a reward) are provided to an exerciser for the time spent exercising and a criterion (e.g., amount of daily exercise time) is indicated to the exerciser as a requirement for earning the rest consequence. In the changing-criterion design, the required level of a target variable is altered repeatedly (e.g., increasing the amount of daily exercise time) to improve performance of this variable over time. Indeed, the effects of an intervention are demonstrated when the target variable (e.g., behaviour) changes in relation to the presentation of a criterion (Kinugasa et al. 2004).

The changing-criterion design has a number of important characteristics. First, unlike A–B–A–B designs, changing-criterion designs typically do not require the withdrawal of an intervention to allow researchers and practitioners to ascertain intervention effectiveness (although some variations of the design include a withdrawal phase). Second, unlike multiple-baseline designs, the intervention is not applied to one behaviour and then eventually to others, or it is temporarily withheld for various baselines. In short, the changing-criterion design does not withdraw or withhold interventions to demonstrate treatment effectiveness (Kazdin 1982). Also, unlike the A–B–A–B design and the multiple-baseline design, which can be applied to psychological constructs (e.g., confidence), or outcomes (performance), the changing-criterion design is really only suitable for behaviours. It is difficult to devise an intervention that increases psychological constructs in the stepwise controlled manner required by the changing-criterion design.

The changing-criterion design is a 'within-series' procedure, thus allowing threats to internal validity to be ruled out by bringing the level of the dependent variable under the control of certain criteria that are modified during a study (Hall and Fox 1977; Hartmann and Hall 1976). Typically, in this design a baseline phase (phase A) is used, which is followed by an intervention phase (phase B); this is then implemented continually for a period of time until criterion performance is achieved (e.g., an increase in minutes of daily exercise). At certain selected points during the intervention phase, stepwise changes in the level of the performance on the dependent variable are implemented (phase B). Moreover, certain criteria are linked with treatment contingencies and, if the dependent measure generally follows the stepwise change in the preset criteria, validity for a treatment effect is enhanced (Kazdin 1982; Kratochwill et al. 1984). To illustrate, imagine that, like Bill in our case example earlier in this chapter, a person has been instructed by their GP to undertake regular exercise for health reasons. The collection of baseline data indicated that the prevalence of daily exercise (in minutes) for this person is zero. Therefore, the exercise psychologist working with the person prescribes an intervention that consists of setting the criterion of exercising for fifteen minutes a day, five times a week. In addition, the exercise psychologist includes a condition whereby if the criterion is met or exceeded (fifteen minutes or more of daily exercise) the person will earn a reinforcing consequence (e.g., money vouchers towards an iPod). This type of design is very much like a goal-setting intervention and therefore is likely to be effective because reaching criterion is motivational and also provides structure (Latham and Locke 2002). Monitoring of whether the criterion is met or not is undertaken and recorded daily by the exercise psychologist; when daily exercise meets or exceeds the criterion, the person is provided with the vouchers. In addition, when the criterion is met for several days, the bar is raised slightly (e.g., twenty minutes a day, five times a week). Following the stabilization of performance at this new level, the criterion is again increased to another level (e.g., twenty-five minutes a day, five times a week). This pattern (i.e., increases in the criterion) continues until a desired level of the target variable (e.g., exercise) is attained.

Figure 7.1 highlights how these data might look if presented in graphical form. In essence, the baseline phase is followed by an intervention phase, and several subphases of the intervention are indicated by dashed vertical lines. In each subphase the new criterion for exercise is identified by horizontal dashed lines.

The rationale for the changing-criterion design is largely similar to that underlying those designs already presented in this book. First, the baseline allows one to describe current and predict future target variables (e.g., behaviour). Second, the subphases of the intervention allow for the making and testing of predictions about intervention effectiveness. To illustrate, because each subphase has a new criterion, if the intervention is responsible for any change in behaviour, then behaviour would be expected to follow the changes in the criterion. Therefore, random fluctuations in behaviour that deviate away from increases in the criterion are more likely to be because of extraneous variables rather than the specific intervention (Kazdin 1982).

The changing-criterion design is most appropriate for evaluating the effects of interventions that aim to change (i.e., accelerate or decelerate) one target behaviour of one participant in a systematic stepwise format (i.e., gradually shaping). Accordingly, these designs have been used to bring about changes in behaviour

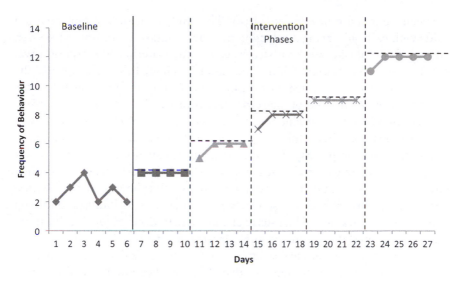

FIGURE 7.1 Hypothetical data from a changing-criterion design containing several subphases during the intervention.

across a variety of domains (see McDougall, Hawkins, Brady and Jenkins 2006). Moreover, they have proved typically useful in relation to studying intervention effectiveness on long-standing, habitual behaviours. These behaviours include, for example, smoking reduction (Edinger 1978; Hartmann and Hall 1976; Weis and Hall 1971), excessive coffee drinking (Foxx and Rubinoff 1979), separation anxiety (Flood and Wilder 2004), medical regimen compliance (Gorski and Westbrook 2004), food acceptance (Kahng, Boscoe and Byrne 2003; Luiselli 2000), leisure-time reading in schizophrenic adults (Skinner, Skinner and Armstrong 2000), work rate in adults with severe mental retardation (Bates, Renzaglia and Clees 1980), exercise frequency in obese children (DeLuca and Holborn 1992), bike riding in a child with Asperger's syndrome (Cameron, Shapiro and Ainsleigh 2005), excessive blood glucose monitoring (Allen and Evans 2001), successful completion of maths problems in children (Hall and Fox 1977), treatment for obsessive-compulsive disorder (Arco 2008) and autism (Ganz and Flores 2008, 2009).

The rest of this section provides three examples of the changing-criterion design and illustrates how the design can be used to reduce, enhance and shape behaviour. First, Foxx and Rubinoff (1979) used the changing-criterion design to evaluate the effects of a programme for individuals who consumed large amounts of caffeine in their daily diets (i.e., reduce behaviour). More specifically, the intervention (presented to three participants) comprised a monetary reinforcement procedure in which participants had to deposit $20 which would be returned in small portions if they fell below the criterion for the maximum level of caffeine that could be consumed on a particular day. At baseline, all three participants consumed a daily caffeine intake of more than 1,000 mg (i.e., between eight and nine cups of coffee). The study consisted of four criterion shifts with each shift being a reduction in caffeine intake by 100 mg. Moreover, when caffeine intake was consistently below the criterion, the criterion was reduced by approximately 100 mg less then baseline. In each subphase, the money reinforcer was earned only if caffeine consumption fell at or below the criterion level. At the end of the study, data revealed that all three participants had reduced their daily caffeine consumption to less than 600 mg per day (fewer than five cups of coffee), while two participants had reduced their consumption to less than 400 mg per day. The study further revealed that the intervention effect was maintained for almost a year with all three participants consuming fewer than five cups of coffee per day at a ten-month follow-up data collection phase. Again, this study demonstrates the importance of including a follow-up to demonstrate meaningful long-term change in behaviour. Figure 7.2 illustrates the reduction in caffeine consumption for participant 1.

A second advantage of the changing-criterion design is that it can be used to instil or enhance new behaviours so that they may become habitual in a participant's behavioural repertoire (Kinugasa et al. 2004). To illustrate, DeLuca

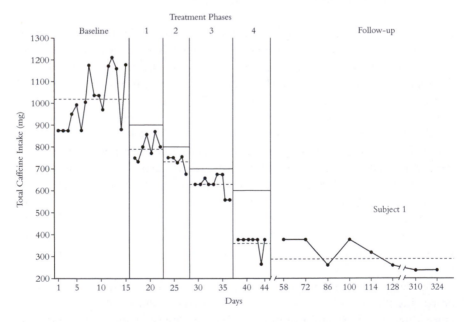

FIGURE 7.2 Subject's daily caffeine intake (mg) during baseline, treatment and follow-up. The criterion level for each treatment phase was 102 mg of caffeine less than the previous treatment phase. Solid horizontal lines indicate the criterion level for each phase. Broken horizontal lines indicate the mean for each condition. Adapted with permission from R. M. Foxx and A. Rubinoff (1979) Behavioral treatment of caffeinism: Reducing excessive coffee drinking. *Journal of Applied Behavior Analysis, 12*, 335–344.

and Holborn (1992) used a changing-criterion design to increase the amount of exercise undertaken in six obese and non-obese boys. The participants rode stationary bikes and received feedback (i.e., a light illuminated and a bell rang) when they worked as hard as the criterion specified and performed the required number of rotations of the exercise bike wheel. At baseline, measures for the participants were taken on the dependent variable of number of wheel rotations. During the intervention, the participants adhered to three criterion shifts in which they had to increase their bike riding by 15 per cent above their average performance in the previous condition. Following the three criterion increases, a return to baseline was scheduled as a check on the experimental manipulation. Data revealed that all of the participants increased their wheel rotations in correspondence with the criterion shifts (i.e., they exercised harder), and decreases in behaviour were also noted when the conditions were returned to baseline (i.e., criteria were removed).

Finally, because the changing-criterion design contains a stepwise feature (i.e., criterion shift) this provides an opportunity for researchers and practitioners to assess the effectiveness of interventions that teach or shape behaviour (Morgan and Morgan 2009). For example, Cameron et al. (2005) reported using a changing-criterion design over sixty-four sessions with a nine-year-old boy with Asperger's syndrome (a developmental syndrome characterized by social awkwardness) to develop the skill of bicycle riding. The boy had previously attempted to learn to ride his bike but because of failure he had suffered embarrassment and pain. His parents wished him to learn to ride his bike because of the physical and social benefits. Accordingly, an eight-step task analysis was introduced in which initially the participant was instructed and guided through incremental movements related to bike riding. In this initial phase of the intervention the bike was mounted on a stationary training device to allow the participant to master the key skills essential to bike riding (e.g., pedalling, mounting and dismounting). Following the development of these key skills the bike was removed from the training stand and the intervention continued outside. Accordingly, over the phase changes the participant was encouraged to demonstrate an increased percentage mastery of one of the steps in the task analysis for a set duration (e.g., ride for eight minutes, brake and dismount). As a reinforcer the participant was allowed access to his video console when the criteria were met. During the study, the time constraints for each of the phases were gradually increased, along with the inclusion of additional criteria. Data from the study are presented in Figure 7.3 and indicate that cycling time and frequency increased with the presentation of gradual and small criterion increments across the study. Overall, the eight-step task analysis facilitated the participant's ability to ride his bike across a 0.5-km distance. Moreover, a two-week follow-up revealed that the participant was continuing in his bike riding and even took part in an 8-km fundraising ride.

The three preceding examples highlight the flexible nature of the changing-criterion design in assessing intervention effectiveness in relation to reducing,

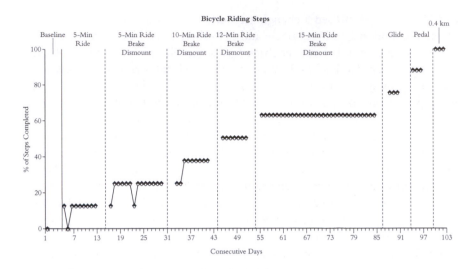

FIGURE 7.3 The filled diamonds depict the percentage of the eight-step task analysis that was completed during a session. Condition labels appear between condition lines. Adapted with permission from M. J. Cameron, R. L. Shapiro and S. A. Ainsleigh (2005) Bicycle riding: Pedalling made possible through behavioral interventions. *Journal of Positive Behavior Interventions,* 7, 153–158.

enhancing or shaping behaviour. For an intervention to be concluded as affecting performance, various criteria must be met in relation to the target behaviour within each phase change or change in criterion, and behaviour must exceed or stay below the criterion (Hartmann and Hall 1976). To illustrate, interventions may be devised using a changing-criterion design that aim to increase or reduce the prevalence of a particular behaviour. The following section explores examples of the changing-criterion design from the sport and exercise literature.

The changing-criterion design in sport and exercise: illustrations

Although the popularity of the changing-criterion design in mainstream applied psychology research is well documented (McDougall et al. 2006), this design remains rare in the sport research literature (Kinugasa et al. 2004). In contrast, evidence of changing-criterion designs being applied in exercise settings is more prevalent, with many examples using exercise settings or interventions to enhance exercise-related behaviours (see Cameron et al. 2005; DeLuca and Holborn 1992). Despite the paucity of specific sport examples, the domains of education (e.g., Ganz and Flores 2008, 2009), and more specifically physical education, and coaching provide some illustrations of this design. For example, Rush and Ayllon (1984) compared the effects of conventional coaching and peer behavioural coaching on the performance of a series of soccer skills (i.e., heading, throw-ins, and goal kicks) in nine boys aged from eight to ten years from the same club using a multiple-baseline design, a reversal design and a changing-criterion design. The nine players were observed twice a week during regular soccer practice sessions for six weeks. Each session lasted for approximately ninety minutes, during which each player was observed for twelve to eighteen trials for each of the three soccer skills. Each skill was observed and defined in terms of outcome. The peer behavioural coaching required a twelve-year-old assistant at the club to coach those players who were having problems on the three skills. Specifically, the peer behavioural coaching intervention comprised the following routine: (1) the players execute the skills and the peer coach judges their performance, (2) the peer coach models the correct skill and (3) the players imitate the correct skill. The changing-criterion design was used for the skill of throw-ins with two players who had not improved their throwing of the ball to the target area after initially using a reversal design in which standard coaching and behavioural coaching were alternated across four phases. Therefore, for these two players the distance to the target area was initially halved down to 3.03 m and then gradually increased back to the full distance of 6.06 m through criterion shifts. Data revealed the shaping process and the use of criterion shifts facilitated a gradual change in the players' throw-in performance.

In addition to its use in physical education and coaching settings, the changing-criterion design has been postulated to assist the achievement of athletes' goals (Kinugasa et al. 2004). For example, when a cricket fast bowler who can bowl at 140 km/hour wants to increase his bowling speed to 150 km/hour, a coach initially sets an improvement of 2 km/hour as a target and provides a financial incentive as a reward. Then a specific strength-training programme is initiated for the bowler until he reaches the speed of 142 km/hour. Following the stabilization of speeds at this criterion, a new criterion (i.e., 144 km/hour) is set along with adjustments being made to the strength programme and presentation of a further financial incentive. This process is then repeated until the bowler reaches his goal of 150 km/hour. Figure 7.4 provides a graphical representation of these data showing that bowling speeds increase with the presentation of each criterion until the desired speed is attained.

Overall, the changing-criterion design is probably the *least used* single-case research design in applied sport and exercise psychology (Hrycaiko and Martin 1996). This situation could be because of a lack of awareness of the benefits of this design by researchers and practitioners in the field (Kinugasa et al. 2004). However, another explanation for the dearth of its usage is that because the design is restricted to enhancing, reducing or shaping changes in habitual behaviour (e.g., Kazdin 1982) it may be deemed less appropriate for sport and exercise. For example, participants are often not after gradual changes in behaviour, but rather are keen to eliminate undesirable behaviours or maximize desirable behaviours in as short a time frame as possible. Therefore, researchers and practitioners may consider adopting the changing-criterion design in situations in which it

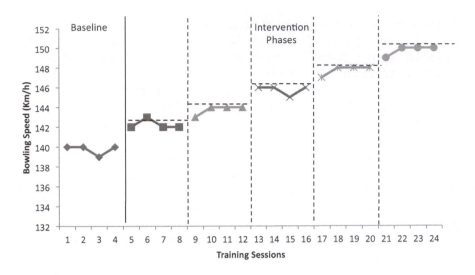

FIGURE 7.4 Hypothetical data from a changing-criterion design used to increase the bowling speeds of a cricket fast bowler.

is important to bring about gradual changes in important exercise and sport behaviours (e.g., exercise adherence and skill development).

Design variations

Because the changing-criterion design has generally been underused by researchers and practitioners in comparison with other single-case designs, very few variations of the design have been created (McDougall, Smith, Black and Rumrill 2005). Most applications of the design have followed the basic design illustrated in the previous section with subtle variations in relation to the number of changes that are made in the criterion (i.e., the number of subphases) and the length of the subphases under each criterion (i.e., the number of observations). Recently, researchers have developed and applied two variations of the basic changing-criterion design (McDougall 2005, 2006; McDougall et al. 2006). The following sections explore these variations along with their suitability for sport and exercise settings.

The range-bound changing-criterion design

In sport and exercise settings it may be appropriate to place certain constraints on a participant following the presentation of an intervention to protect their well-being. To illustrate, if an injured athlete is undergoing an exercise rehabilitation programme it is essential that they do not overtrain and therefore increase the likelihood of re-injury. Accordingly, in this situation the practitioner may wish to restrict the amount of exercise that the athlete is undertaking, and the range-bound changing-criterion (RBCC) design modification is pertinent for this situation (McDougall 2005). Essentially, the RBCC design is a simple variation of the classic changing-criterion design and comprises upper and lower limits for each criterion that is prescribed. In this design the target behaviour must match or exceed the lower performance criterion and concurrently match or be less than the higher performance criterion. Success is achieved when a participant's behaviour resides within or conforms to the stipulated range criterion (e.g., exercise at least four times per week, but no more than five; McDougall et al. 2006). The RBCC design includes a baseline followed by a series of intervention phases, each of which has a stepwise changing criterion for performance and serves as a baseline for subsequent phases of the intervention (McDougall et al. 2006). This design is applicable to situations in which an acceleration or a deceleration of target behaviours is required. It also lends itself to the shaping of behaviour (Alberto and Troutman 1999), cognitive-behavioural modification (Kottler 2001) and behavioural self-management procedures (e.g., self-monitoring, self-verbalization and self-evaluation; McDougall 1998). An example of this design is found in McDougall (2005), who used an RBCC design with an obese man who wished to gradually increase the time he spent running. Following the collection of baseline data, the practitioner decided that an initial running time of twenty minutes should be set for the first criterion. Typically, in the basic changing-criterion design a time exceeding twenty minutes would have met the criterion; however, in the RBCC variation a range of running durations (i.e., upper and lower limits) is prescribed. Moreover, it has been recommended that this range be around 10 per cent (McDougall 2005). With regard to the current example, the man was presented with a running limit for the first criterion of eighteen to twenty-two minutes. The major assumption underlying the range used in this design is that it allows for variability in target behaviour responses and also avoids excessive demonstration of the target behaviour that may be harmful to the participant (e.g., overtraining). Data from the study are illustrated in Figure 7.5. This figure shows that the man's running time increased from twenty to 100 minutes with running times staying within the 10 per cent range throughout the study.

Another important facet of the RBCC design is that the criterion can be relaxed or reverted back to an earlier, easier criterion at any point during the study. Indeed, relaxing the criterion provides an opportunity for rest and recovery from the constant challenge of continuous improvement. Although returning behaviour to an earlier criterion provides an opportunity to establish the internal validity of the intervention (e.g., if a participant's behaviour tracks the new lower criterion it is unlikely that the target behaviour was attributable to extraneous variables, particularly when increases are demonstrated with the presentation of a new criterion; McDougall et al. 2006). An example of this reversal phase is demonstrated in the fifth phase change in Figure 7.5.

Overall, the RBCC design is a simple variation of the classic changing-criterion design. The main difference between the two designs concerns the

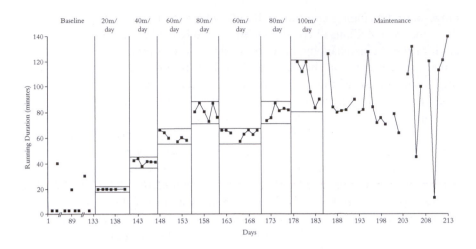

FIGURE 7.5 Duration, in minutes, of daily exercise (i.e., running) during the baseline, intervention and maintenance phases. Note: Baseline is truncated to permit display of all data from intervention and maintenance phases. Participant ran on three days during the nineteen-week baseline phase. Parallel horizontal lines within the seven intervention phases depict performance criteria that participant established for self to define the range of acceptable performance for each phase. Upper horizontal line indicates the maximum number of minutes of running permitted, lower horizontal line indicates the minimum number of minutes of running permitted. Adapted with permission from D. McDougall (2005) The range-bound changing criterion design. *Behavioral Interventions, 20*, 132. Wiley and Sons.

specification of a bounded range of expected performance rather than a single point criterion. Typically, this range is defined by an upper and lower limit following the collection of baseline. Finally, the RBCC design provides an opportunity for establishing the internal validity of an intervention through the relaxing or reverting of criteria (McDougall 2005). Currently, there is no evidence of an RBCC design being used in the sport literature – although the RBCC has been presented as being applicable to exercise given that it is entirely consistent with well-known principles of physical exercise (see McDougall et al. 2006). The following section describes a further new modification to the changing-criterion design.

The distributed-criterion design

A further recent design innovation to the changing-criterion design is the distributed-criterion (DC) design (McDougall 2006; McDougall et al. 2006; McDougall and Smith 2006). The DC design is typically used to evaluate the effects of interventions for one target behaviour occurring in the same or different environments (e.g., self-confidence across training and competition), or several target behaviours occurring in the same or different environments (e.g., effort and enjoyment across training and competition). The design is accordingly suited to studies investigating 'multi-tasking' strategies in which individuals allocate time to numerous interdependent tasks conducted at the same time or in the same contexts in ways that relate to changing environmental demands (Morgan and Morgan 2009; McDougall et al. 2006). For example, a person diagnosed with heart disease may be encouraged to adopt a healthier lifestyle involving dedicating time and effort to healthy eating, stress management and exercise. The DC design comprises elements from other single-case designs (i.e., changing-criterion, multiple-baseline and A–B–A–B designs) covered earlier in the book. To illustrate, McDougall et al. (2006) has indicated that in the DC design there are concurrent baselines across three contexts or behaviours, a series of concurrent intervention phases (changing-criterion features), multiple-target behaviours or contexts (multiple-baseline design features) and a reversal phase (A–B–A–B features). In the DC design, experimental control is determined when the target behaviour conforms quickly, precisely and in a stable fashion to changes in the criterion across the sequential intervention phases. Experimental control is enhanced when the interdependent target behaviours conform simultaneously to changes in criterion that are distributed across concurrent intervention phases. The DC design is therefore most applicable to evaluating interventions that aim to change concurrently (by way of small- or large-level changes and in two directions) interdependent behaviour across multiple settings (McDougall et al. 2006).

Currently, the only intervention study in applied research using a DC design is that by McDougall (2006). The participant (an academic researcher) used goal-setting and multiple behavioural management components in an effort to increase research productivity. 'Productivity' was defined as the mean number of minutes that the participant spent performing activities to complete three journal manuscripts for submission to professional journals (e.g., analysing data, drafting charts, writing and editing). During baseline, the participant self-recorded research productivity for each of the three manuscripts (A, B and C). During the intervention phases, the participant continued to self-record but also used goal-setting (e.g., establishing dates by which the manuscripts had to be completed) and self-graphing (e.g., posting research activity on a line graph). The overall criterion for the participant's total productivity within and across all intervention phases was fixed at a mean of three hours per day, while the productivity criteria for each of the three manuscripts were varied. To illustrate, the three hours of work time across the three manuscripts were distributed in accordance with the multi-tasking nature of the intervention and target behaviour. Productivity criteria for each manuscript were shifted in line with the participant's need to vary the amount of time spent working on the manuscripts because of the manuscripts being at various stages of development (e.g., initial drafts, nearly complete, complete). These distributed-criteria lines are illustrated in Figure 7.6. Furthermore, the prescribed time requirements were eliminated for a manuscript when a stage of completion was reached. Indeed, this phase of the study served as a reversal aspect. Overall, data illustrated in Figure 7.6 demonstrate a substantial increase in overall productivity in comparison with baseline levels. In addition, allotted time requirements were met during each phase change, and time was differentially allocated to the manuscripts when appropriate (e.g., different stages of completion).

The internal validity of an intervention in the DC design is established when a number of key observations are noted. For example, inferences regarding *intervention effectiveness* are made when sequential (i.e., across adjacent phases) and concurrent (i.e., across behaviours or contexts) changes in the target behaviour and bidirectional changes in target behaviour (i.e., both increases and decreases) are noted, and when phase changes correspond to meaningful changes in the target behaviour (McDougall 2006).

The DC design is the newest addition to the changing-criterion design and incorporates elements of the changing-criterion, multiple-baseline and A–B–A–B designs. In the DC design, experimental control is typically demonstrated through numerous replications and the distinctiveness of the design makes it appealing to evaluate experimental control in studies that target interdependent performance in ever-changing, multi-tasking situations. The DC design may be appropriate for athletes who must alter the intensity, duration and type of training relative to their goals and to prepare them for competitions spread across a season. Because of the design requirements (i.e., multi-tasking situations), the DC is more complex and thus has received scant research application and attention in the behavioural sciences and sport and exercise specifically (see McDougall 2006; McDougall et al. 2006). Despite the lack of application the DC remains a worthwhile innovation and addition to the single-case method.

Interim summary

The changing-criterion design is particularly useful for assessing intervention effectiveness on target behaviours that are likely to change gradually over time (e.g., skill acquisition, exercise adherence). Typically, in the changing-criterion design, baseline measurement of the target behaviours takes place, following which a series of phase changes is facilitated through the presentation of criteria pertinent to the target behaviour. This may involve target behaviour being increased (e.g., exercise adherence) or decreased (e.g., alcohol intake) depending on the aims of the programme (e.g., healthy lifestyle). Causal inferences about intervention effectiveness are determined in this design when changes in the target behaviour relative to set criteria are observed across three or more phases. The RBCC and DC represent the most recent innovations to the changing-criterion design. The development of these designs reflects the appraisal by practitioners to determine intervention effectiveness with participants governed

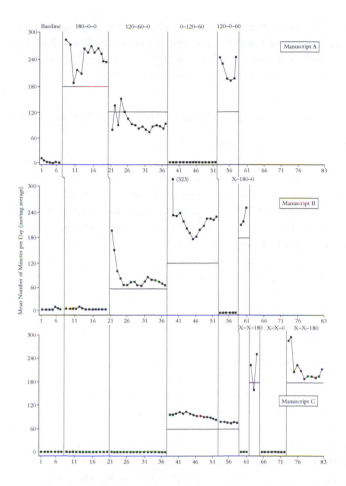

FIGURE 7.6 Moving average for research productivity (mean number of minutes expended daily) within baseline and intervention phases for Manuscripts A, B and C. Note: Horizontal lines indicate within-phase productivity criteria (i.e., minimum number of minutes to be expended on manuscript) that participant set for self. Labels for intervention phases appear as numeric sequences (e.g., 120–60–0), with the first numeral indicating the within-phase criterion (mean number of minutes) that the participant established for Manuscript A, the second numeral indicating the within-phase criterion for Manuscript B and the third numeral indicating the within-phase criterion for Manuscript C. X indicates that a criterion was no longer pertinent because the participant had completed work on that manuscript. From 'The Distributed Criterion Design', by D. McDougall, in press, *Journal of Behavioral Education.* Copyright 2005 by Springer-Verlag. Adapted with permission from D. McDougall, J. Hawkins, M. Brady and A. Jenkins (2006) Recent innovations in the changing criterion design: Implications for research and practice in special education. *Journal of Special Education, 40,* 2–15.

by ranges in behaviour and those in multi-tasking situations where there are likely to be large variations in behaviour across individuals (McDougall 2005). To date, there is scant evidence of the RBCC and DC being used in applied behavioural research, and sport and exercise specifically.

Problems and limitations of the changing-criterion design

Typically, issues regarding the relationship between behaviour and changes in criteria have been identified and form the backbone of changing-criterion limitations (Kazdin 1982). First, the strength of the changes in behaviour as a consequence of a criterion shift depends largely on the close correspondence between the criterion and behaviour during an intervention. However, in reality it is unlikely that the level of behaviour being assessed will fall exactly in line with each criterion level and therefore this may cause ambiguity regarding the intervention accounting for change in the target behaviour. In cases in which correspondence is not close, researchers may refer to mean levels of behaviour across the intervention subphases to demonstrate a stepwise relationship. Second, another important factor contributing to a lack of correspondence between criterion and behaviour is that, when the intervention is first presented, behaviour is likely to change rapidly, with any improvements likely to exceed the first target criterion. This is problematic because the changing-criterion design is based around facilitating gradual changes in behaviour (e.g., shaping), not rapid changes. This limitation further enhances the strength of the RBCC design. Moreover, without drawing from the features of other designs (e.g., reversal phase), it may be difficult to draw causal inferences about rapid changes in behaviour. Third, the number of criterion shifts is an important aspect of the changing-criterion design, with a minimum of two subphases being pertinent to draw causal inferences. If two or more subphases are presented, changes in behaviour can be confidently matched to changes in criterion shifts. Typically, in research more subphases are used to demonstrate intervention effectiveness; however, this is often to the detriment of strong conclusions. For example, when criteria are altered it is important to maintain behaviour at a stable rate at or near the level of the new criterion, otherwise it is difficult to conclude that the criterion and behaviour are related. Researchers using multiple criterion shifts are best served by the criterion level being in effect for a longer period of time to see if the level really influences behaviour. Finally, in the changing-criterion design changes in criteria are made to bring about changes in target behaviours. However, no guidelines exist regarding what the magnitude of change in each criterion should be. Typically, changes in criteria are a reflection of participants' problems and their ability to meet the changes presented to them. To this end, Kazdin (1982) recommended gradual, modest changes in criteria, along with using smaller criterion changes at the start of an intervention to allow participants to maximize their potential.

Although the above limitations may also apply to the RBCC and DC design variations, both designs have a number of additional weaknesses (McDougall et al. 2006). Because the RBCC design can accommodate temporary reversals of direction in target variables, the researcher or practitioner must be considerate of the ethical, practical and experimental reasons for doing so. Indeed, it is possible that reverting behaviour criteria provides a break for participants and bolsters the opportunity for developing short-term and long-term improvements in target behaviour. In contrast, it is also equally likely that reversals in direction of performance criteria could also stagnate change and prolong the time needed to achieve the desired target behaviour. In addition, because the RBCC design is based on the gradual progression of target behaviours (like the changing-criterion design) it is not conducive to interventions that are expected to produce large, immediate changes in target behaviours (Hartmann and Hall 1976; Schloss, Sedlak, Elliot and Smothers 1982). Finally, because of its design requirements, the DC is a more complex design and thus the extent to which it can be applied is limited (McDougall et al. 2006).

Evaluation of the design

Overall, the changing-criterion design (including RBCC and DC variations) contains several features that make it clinically and methodologically sound. The design does not require interventions to be withdrawn or withheld for baseline data collection. Conclusive demonstrations regarding intervention effectiveness are provided when behaviour in the intervention phases matches closely shifts in criteria. One of the more prominent features of the design is the gradual progression towards a desired level in target behaviours (e.g., regular exercise). Accordingly, this feature makes the design applicable to shaping behaviour situations. A key element of the design is ensuring correspondence between changes in behaviour and criteria to determine intervention effectiveness.

Summary

The changing-criterion design (and variations) requires a demonstration of changes in the dependent measure along with criterion shifts over the intervention phase. To establish the internal validity of the design one must demonstrate that each criterion shift results in a change in behaviour (Foxx and Rubinoff 1979). In addition, behaviour must stabilize in the within-phase data before proceeding to the next stepwise level. Furthermore, each stepwise criterion change must be large enough to distinguish it from variability occurring in the data (e.g., see Chapter 5 on behavioural cyclicity; Kratochwill et al. 1984). Procedures within the changing-criterion design include randomly varying the length in the criterion, as well as the magnitude, and the direction of the criterion shifts (Hayes 1981). These procedures can increase inference for experimental control in the design because they help to exaggerate the influence of the criterion shifts (Kratochwill et al. 1984). Overall, the changing-criterion design is useful when shaping behaviour gradually over an intervention or treatment phase is needed. For more complex situations the RBCC and DC represent important innovations to the standard changing-criterion design although limited application of these variations exists in the applied behavioural research. The following chapter outlines a final single-case research design – the alternating-treatments design – which allows researchers and practitioners to assess multiple treatment effects.

Key points

- The changing-criterion design is a single-case research design that includes a baseline phase followed by several intervention phases in which the target behaviour must reach or exceed behavioural criteria as agreed between the practitioner and participant.
- A criterion shift is when gradual increases in the desired target behaviour across the intervention phases are facilitated.
- The range-bound criterion design is a relatively new addition to the changing-criterion design in which target behaviour must fall within a specified range during each intervention phase before criteria are subsequently increased.
- The distributed-criterion design is also a relatively new variation of the changing-criterion design that integrates features from the original, multiple-baseline and withdrawal designs.

Guided study

Based on your reading of Chapter 7 please take some time to respond to the following review questions:

- How does the changing-criterion design differ from the withdrawal and multiple-baseline designs?
- Discuss why the changing-criterion design is applicable to gradual changes in behaviour.
- Explain the limitations of the changing-criterion design.
- Why does the RBCC design offer greater experimental control in determining causal inferences regarding intervention effectiveness?
- Explain the value of the DC design as an addition to the changing-criterion design.
- Explain how internal validity is determined in the changing-criterion design and RBCC and DC variations.

8

THE ALTERNATING-TREATMENTS DESIGN IN SPORT AND EXERCISE

In this chapter, we shall:

*   outline the rationale underlying the use of alternating-treatments designs in sport and exercise;
*   outline variations of the alternating-treatments design;
*   provide guidance on using this design in applied sport and exercise contexts.

CASE EXAMPLE

Eric is an eighteen-year-old tennis player who despite his natural technical skill lacks the necessary mental skills to deal with pressure and maintain confidence and concentration during tournament play. Despite his apparent lack of mental skills, Eric is motivated to be successful in tennis and regularly participates in an intensive training regime. However, when asked to undertake tasks (by his coach) that require independence (e.g., keeping a reflective training diary) Eric often struggles with the challenge and forgets to complete the tasks. Based on recommendations from his coach, Eric has recently undertaken work with a sport psychologist in an effort to improve his mental skills in tennis (using positive self-talk, imagery and goal-setting). The sport psychologist, although pleased with Eric's mental skills development, is somewhat concerned by his lack of motivation in practising his mental skills in his own time.

Introduction and basic rationale for the design

Applied behavioural researchers and practitioners are increasingly expected to draw upon evidence-based practice when using interventions with clients or client groups (e.g., Barlow et al. 2009; Hemmings and Holder 2009). To this end, interventions must be selected by practitioners on the basis that research has deemed them effective relative to a particular issue and/or client or group. Traditionally, nomothetic (see also Chapters 1 and 10) research paradigms have been adopted to identify effective interventions in which large-group studies are used to draw inferences about participants' reactions (e.g., mean responses of a treatment group are compared with mean responses of a control group; Barker et al. 2010). In these research paradigms, comparisons are made between groups and hence inferences about individuals are extrapolations from group data. There are many benefits of using nomothetic research designs. For example, such designs permit the development of principles, laws or global understanding, allow for prediction and have high external validity (Clark-Carter 2009). However, nomothetic research designs often mask individual reactions and responses to interventions (i.e., idiosyncrasies), information that is important to practitioners and researchers working with individual clients and/or client groups. Indeed, this information is often important for the development of the intervention protocol (Hanton and Jones 1999) as well as making conclusions about intervention efficacy and effectiveness (Seligman 1995). Typically, the researcher and practitioner in applied settings is not interested in comparing mean scores from treatment and control groups but is concerned with an individual's response to an intervention over time. Therefore, single-case designs are attractive options to applied investigators because they enable *individual* reactions and responses to be studied through intra-subject, time-series comparison (Kazdin 1982).

A common feature of applied settings is the fact that, whereas a given intervention may work for one client, it may not work for another – and hence an alternative intervention programme may have to be prescribed. Therefore, identifying effective interventions in applied research may also involve comparing treatments (Barlow et al. 2009). For example, when a practitioner has identified (through baseline measures) the target variable to be treated, guidance is often taken from an array of literature supporting more than one potential intervention strategy relative to the target variable. In this instance, the practitioner may take a pragmatic view and choose to use two treatments (both of which are supported in the literature) to see which is more effective (i.e., to which the participant responds best). In single-case terms, this type of design is described as an alternating-treatments design (ATD). In this chapter we first consider the main tenets of the ATD before exploring examples from the literature. We then consider ATD design variations before providing an overall critique of the design.

The ATD design (first described by Barlow and Hayes 1979) involves systematically alternating two or more interventions across time and comparing relative responses of the target variable to each intervention (Kratochwill et al. 1984). Moreover, the ATD allows a participant to be exposed to separate treatment conditions for equal periods of time. To this end the ATD has been defined (Barlow and Hayes 1979) as a between-series design because one is comparing results from two or more separate series of data points. In the ATD, treatments are alternated for a brief period (e.g., treatment A is administered in one session and treatment B in another session). Alternation of the treatments is established by either counterbalancing or randomly assigning treatments across phases of the study (Barlow and Hayes 1979).

The ATD design originates from a group of experimental designs common to the study of operant behaviour in applied settings. These designs include the multiple-schedule design (Hersen and Barlow 1976; Leitenberg 1973), simultaneous-treatment design (Kazdin and Hartmann 1978) and the multi-element design (Ulman and Sulzer-Azaroff 1975) and were used to identify relationships between behaviour and stimulus events in learning experiments (e.g., McGonigle, Rojahn, Dixon and Strain 1987). These designs share the feature of rapidly changing experimental conditions with similar stimuli associated with different conditions. As we will see in the forthcoming sections, the ATD is an extremely flexible and adaptable design, sharing many features with other single-case designs already described in this book. Interestingly, the collection of baseline data is not a requirement of the design (because of clinical or practical concerns) although, when collected, data serve the same purpose as in previous designs: namely to illustrate the natural state of the target variable and to allow comparison between baseline and treatment responses (Wacker et al. 1990).

Inferences about treatment effectiveness in the ATD are a result of the rapid phase changes that occur as interventions are alternated. Moreover, when variable change tracks the rapid phase or treatment changes (i.e., baseline to treatment, or treatment A to treatment B) a treatment effect is observed, making the effect of extraneous variables unlikely (Barlow and Hayes 1979). To illustrate, you may recall Eric our tennis player from earlier in the chapter who was working with a sport psychologist to develop his mental skills but who was erratic in his adherence to self-practice routines. Remember how the sport psychologist asked Eric to document daily adherence records (i.e., minutes of daily self-practice) for five consecutive days. The daily number of minutes that Eric spent practising his mental skills during the baseline is depicted in the first panel of Figure 8.1. From this figure it is evident that the amount of self-practice fluctuates on a daily basis, thus supporting the sport psychologist's conclusion about Eric's erratic adherence rate to his practice routine. Following baseline, the sport psychologist then introduces two treatments (treatment A: email reminders; treatment B: SMS text alerts) on alternative days during an intervention phase to encourage Eric to practise his mental skills. To illustrate, on day six the sport psychologist sent Eric an email (treatment A) after his morning training session at 10 a.m. to remind him to engage in self-practice.

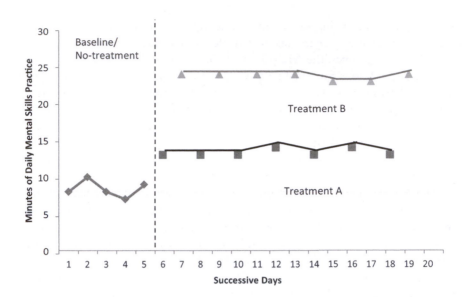

FIGURE 8.1 Hypothetical data from an ATD design containing several subphases during the intervention.

Subsequently, on day seven, the second treatment (B) was instigated in which the sport psychologist sent Eric an SMS text alert following his training session at 10 a.m., again reminding him of his self-practice. These two conditions were then alternated daily for two weeks. These hypothetical data are illustrated in the second panel of Figure 8.1 and demonstrate the amount of time (in minutes) spent engaging in self-practice. Each line in this phase represents adherence to mental skills training under a specific treatment condition, in this case email or text reminders. Interestingly, it is noticeable how data points for each treatment are reported on alternative days and this represents the essence of the ATD design. Overall, the data clearly indicate that treatment B was more effective than treatment A in increasing the amount of time Eric spent self-practising his mental skills. Therefore, in such situations in which the most effective intervention is evident, the practitioner or researcher will often discontinue the least effective treatment and continue a course of intervention involving the effective strategy (Barlow and Hayes 1979).

The use of ATDs in applied research has increased since Kazdin (1982) suggested that they were the least underused single-case design (see Holcombe, Wolery and Gast 1994; Kinugasa et al. 2004; Strømgren and Kolby 1996). The literature now boasts over 700 research reports applying the ATD or design variations comparing the effect of treatment and no treatment (baseline) or comparing two or more distinct treatments (Barlow et al. 2009). The rest of this section provides examples from the literature illustrating these strategies of the ATD.

The research literature contains many examples of studies comparing treatment and no treatment using an ATD (e.g., Jordan, Singh and Repp 1989; O'Brien, Azrin and Henson 1969). Ollendick, Shapiro and Barrett (1981) conducted a notable study using an ATD to compare treatment and no treatment conditions. Specifically, the study compared the effects of two treatments (i.e., physical restraint and positive practice overcorrection) with no treatment (i.e., continued baseline) in the reduction of stereotypic behaviour in three children with severe intellectual disabilities. The target variables of the study involved bizarre hand movements (e.g., hair twirling and hand posturing). The study comprised the administration of three fifteen-minute sessions each day by the same experimenter. Following the collection of baseline data for all three time periods, the two treatments and the no treatment were issued in a counterbalanced manner across the sessions. During the sessions, each participant was positioned at a small table in a classroom and instructed by the experimenter to work on one of several visual motor tasks. Treatment one (physical restraint) consisted of a verbal warning and manual restraint of the participant's hand on the tabletop for thirty seconds on the presentation of the stereotypic behaviour (e.g., hair twirling). Treatment two (positive practice overcorrection) consisted of the same verbal warning but was subsequently followed by manual guidance in appropriate manipulation of the task materials for thirty seconds. The no treatment condition consisted of an extended baseline in which the experimenter monitored behaviour occurrence and task performance. Throughout the study data were collected on the total number of stereotypic behaviours during each session and performance on the visual motor tasks. Importantly, in this study when one of the treatments produced a zero or near-zero rate of stereotypic behaviour that treatment was then selected and presented across all three time periods for the remainder of the study. Data collected from two of the study's participants are illustrated in Figures 8.2 and 8.3. Data collected for John in Figure 8.2 demonstrate physical restraint to be the most effective treatment, whereas, in contrast, data for Tim (Figure 8.3) reveal positive practice to be the most effective.

In contrast to the above illustration of an ATD comparing treatments with no treatment, the following example typifies the common application of the ATD in comparing the relative effects of two or more relevant treatments. To illustrate, in their study Agras, Leitenberg, Barlow and Thomson (1969) evaluated the effects of social reinforcement in the treatment of a fifty-year-old hospitalized women suffering from claustrophobia. This participant was unable to remain in rooms with doors closed, lifts or cinemas, or spend long periods of time in a car. Her fears had intensified following the death of her husband seven years earlier. Baseline data consisted of asking the participant to sit in a small windowless room and monitoring the length of time it took until she became uncomfortable. This process was replicated four times each day (block of trials). Following baseline, the two therapists worked with the participant to help her become more comfortable being in the small windowless room. Typically, each day both

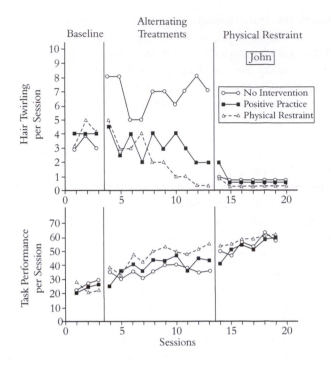

FIGURE 8.2 Stereotypic hair twirling and accurate task performance for John across experimental conditions. The data are plotted across the three alternating time periods according to the schedule that the treatments were in effect. The three treatments, however, were presented only during the alternating-treatments phase. During the last phase, physical restraint was used during all three time periods. Adapted with permission from T. H. Ollendick, E. S. Shapiro, R. P. Barrett (1981) Reducing stereotypic behaviors: An analysis of treatment procedures utilizing an alternating treatments design. *Behavior Therapy, 40*, 570–577.

therapists worked with the participant for two sessions each. One therapist provided praise when the participant increased her time in the room, whereas the other maintained a friendly relationship with the participant without presenting any praise. The ATD, therefore, compared the two treatments of contingent praise versus no praise, and investigated whether or not the participant could discriminate between the different therapist–intervention combinations. Data were collected on the time in seconds that the participant spent in the room across the phases of the study. In the first intervention phase time spent in the small room was increased with the therapist who provided reinforcement (RT) in comparison with the therapist who provided no reinforcement (NRT). In phase two of the intervention the therapists changed roles (i.e., the person who provided RT provided NRT and vice versa) and data indicated that the participant discriminated between the therapists and therefore performance was

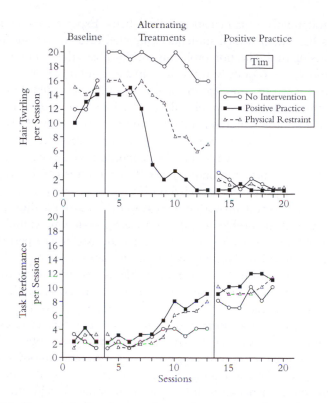

FIGURE 8.3 Stereotypic hand posturing and accurate task performance for Tim across experimental conditions. The data are plotted across the three alternating time periods according to the schedule that the treatments were in effect. The three treatments, however, were presented only during the alternating-treatments phase. During the last phase, positive practice overcorrection restraint was used during all three time periods. Adapted with permission from T. H. Ollendick, E. S. Shapiro, R. P. Barrett (1981) 'Reducing stereotypic behaviors: An analysis of treatment procedures utilizing an alternating treatments design', *Behavior Therapy*, 40: 570–577.

maintained with the therapist providing praise. In the third and final phase the therapists returned to their initial roles and the participant again discriminated between them. In sum, data indicated that the participant remained in the room for *longer* when she consulted with the therapist who provided reinforcement.

Another more recent example of comparing the effects of two or more treatments is provided by Rhymer, Dittmer, Skinner and Jackson (2000), who used an ATD to evaluate the effectiveness of an educational programme that combined timings (using chess clocks), peer tutoring (i.e., peer-delivered immediate feedback), positive practice overcorrection following errors, and performance feedback on mathematics fluency (i.e., speed of accurate responding) in four elementary students with mathematics skills deficits. Experimental conditions consisted of a baseline in which students completed three maths sheets (A, B and C) comprising multiplication problems. In this phase they were instructed to complete the sheets as quickly as possible, in a one-minute time phase. The time in seconds taken to complete the sheets was then recorded. During the intervention phase, students were placed in a dyad and had a chess clock that was set to two minutes. Three sets of multiplication problems (A, B and C) were assigned to one of three conditions (tutee, tutor and control). For example, for student 1, set C was assigned to the tutee condition (i.e., in which students were paired and took turns responding), set B to the tutor condition (i.e., in which students were paired and provided positive practice overcorrection feedback following an incorrect answer) and set A to the control condition (i.e., in which no practice of the problems had taken place). Following completion of the above procedures on five separate occasions, an assessment performance feedback phase was added. Typically, before each maths assessment, students were told their highest number of correct problems per minute regardless of which set of problems was being assessed (A, B or C). Moreover, students were encouraged to try and beat their record during subsequent assessments. Finally, six and seven weeks after the last intervention session, two further assessments were conducted to assess the maintenance effects of the interventions. During these assessments, each set of problems was assessed in random order. Data as illustrated in Figures 8.4 and 8.5 depict the number of problems correct per minute for the four students across the phases of the study. Specifically, the data indicate that serving as tutee and as a tutor, and receiving assessment performance feedback, resulted in initial and maintained increases in maths fluency for three of the four students (1, 3 and 4). In addition, none of the students showed improvement on the control set of problems.

Overall, the ATD is useful and appropriate when a researcher or practitioner is concerned with comparing treatments with no treatment or with comparing two or more treatments with the same participant. Rapidly alternating the treatments allows for multiple comparisons of the target variable(s) responses under different treatment conditions (Holcombe et al. 1994). The illustrations in this section demonstrate how the ATD has been used in applied behavioural research. The following section explores research using the ATD in sport and exercise settings.

The alternating-treatments design in sport and exercise: illustrations

Numerous examples of the ATD can be found in mainstream applied behavioural research (e.g., Barlow et al. 2009); however, in the sport and exercise literature this trend is less obvious (Kinugasa et al. 2004). For example, Hrycaiko and Martin (1996) reported that, since an initial publication in a sport setting by McKenzie and Liskevych (1983) comparing the effects of three different

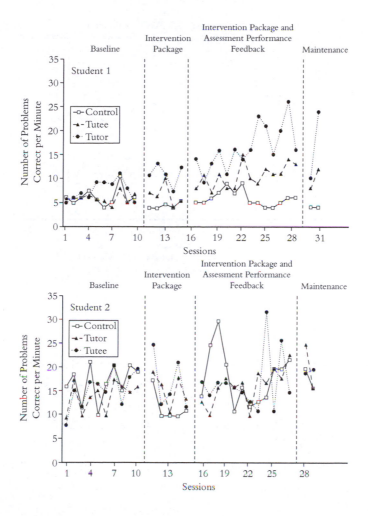

FIGURE 8.4 Number of problems correct per minute for students 1 and 2. From K. N. Rhymer, K. I. Dittmer, C. H. Skinner and B. Jackson (2000) Effectiveness of a multi-component treatment for improving mathematics fluency. *School Psychology Quarterly, 15*, 40–51. American Psychological Association. Adapted with permission.

treatments to improve per cent accuracy of setting in volleyball, not a single article published in the *Journal of Sport and Exercise Psychology* (1979–1994), *The Sport Psychologist* (1987–1994) or *Journal of Applied Sport Psychology* (1989–1994) had used the ATD design. Furthermore, a recent and broader search of the sport and exercise and applied behaviour journals has yielded only a few additional publications of the ATD in the contexts of sport and physical education.

In our first example, Wolko et al. (1993) used an ATD in a sport setting to compare the effects of standard coaching (i.e., baseline condition) with those of standard coaching plus public self-regulation (i.e., self-controlling emotions,

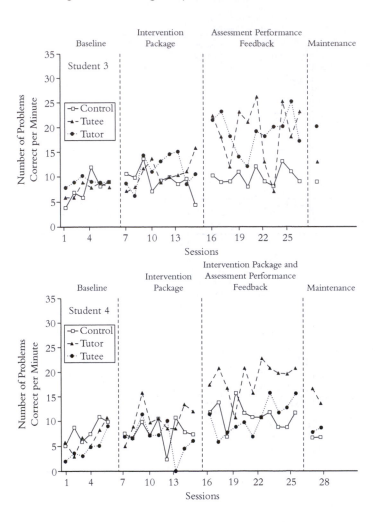

FIGURE 8.5 Number of problems correct per minute for students 3 and 4. From K. N. Rhymer, K. I. Dittmer, C. H. Skinner and B. Jackson (2000) Effectiveness of a multi-component treatment for improving mathematics fluency. *School Psychology Quarterly, 15*, 40–51. American Psychological Association. Adapted with permission.

behaviours and desires; treatment 1), against standard coaching plus private self-regulation (treatment 2) on the frequency of successfully completing gymnastic beam skills (*n* = five gymnasts). Each condition lasted for six sessions, with the conditions being randomly alternated across eighteen sessions. Data presented for one of the gymnasts in Figure 8.6 reveals self-regulation (treatment 2) to be the most effective intervention. Overall, data demonstrated that treatment 2 was more effective than treatment 1 in three of the five gymnasts, whereas one of the gymnasts showed mixed results relative to the effects of the interventions (i.e.,

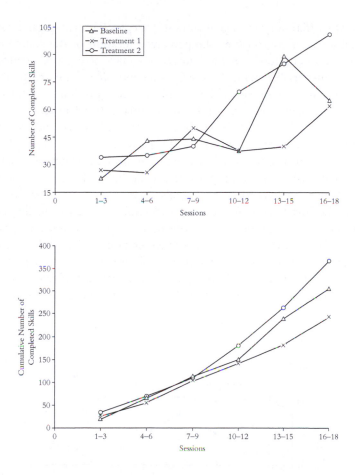

FIGURE 8.6 Frequency of completed beam skills for a gymnast under conditions of standard coaching (baseline), standard coaching plus self-regulation (treatment 1), versus standard coaching plus private self-regulation (treatment 2). Each condition was in effect for six sessions, with the conditions randomly alternating across a total of eighteen sessions. The top panel shows the data plotted as a frequency graph, and the bottom panel shows that same data plotted cumulatively across sessions. This graph was adapted from data presented by Wolko, Hrycaiko and Martin (1993). Adapted from D. Hrycaiko and G. Martin (1996) Applied research studies within single-subject designs: Why so few? *Journal of Applied Sport Psychology, 8,* 183–199 (Taylor & Francis Ltd, http://www. informaworld.com) by permission of the publisher.

treatment 1 was most effective for frequency of attempted skill and treatment 2 was most effective for frequency of completed skill).

A more recent example of the ATD in a sport setting is provided by Lambert, Moore and Dixon (1999). These researchers investigated the relationship between two different types of goal-setting strategies (i.e., self-set and coach-set goals) and locus of control (i.e., the perceived location of the source of control over one's behaviour – namely internal agency or external agency) with the dependent variable being 'on-task' behaviour (e.g., the frequency with which particular exercises would be completed during training sessions on the beam). Four female level eight and nine gymnasts (aged twelve or thirteen) were selected to take part in the study, two with an internal and two with an external locus of control. Using the ATD, participants were exposed to both goal-setting conditions. In the self-set goals condition, participants noted three self-generated goals concerning practice on the beam. In the coach-set goals condition, the coach assigned three goals relative to beam practice without consulting the participants. When clear and stable differences in the data collected under the two treatment conditions became apparent, a second phase was implemented (i.e., after twelve sessions, at which point a clear and stable separation in the data for the two treatments was observed for all four participants, phase two was implemented). In this phase, participants received the treatment that had been shown to be effective in phase one. Overall, data (Figures 8.7 and

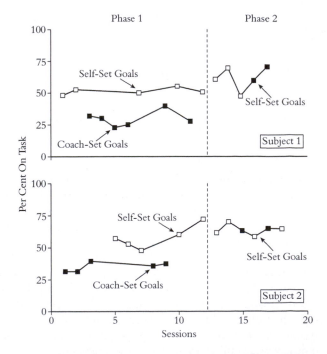

FIGURE 8.7 Per cent on task of participants with an internal locus of control. Adapted from S. M. Lambert, D. W. Moore and R. S. Dixon (1999) Gymnasts in training: The differential effects of self- and coach-set goals as a function of locus of control. *Journal of Applied Sport Psychology, 11,* 72–82 (Taylor & Francis Ltd, http://www.informaworld.com) by permission of the publisher.

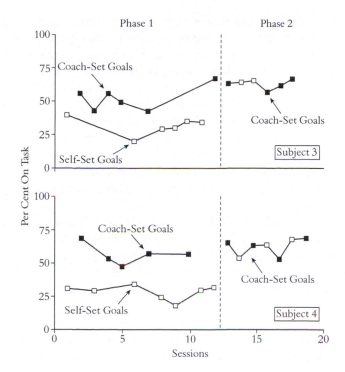

FIGURE 8.8 Per cent on task of participants with an external locus of control. Adapted from S. M. Lambert, D. W. Moore and R. S. Dixon (1999) Gymnasts in training: The differential effects of self- and coach-set goals as a function of locus of control. *Journal of Applied Sport Psychology, 11*, 72–82 (Taylor & Francis Ltd, http://www.informaworld.com) by permission of the publisher.

8.8) revealed differential effects, with participants with a more internal locus of control spending more time on task under the self-set goals condition and those with an external locus of control spending more time on task under coach-set goals. Furthermore, in phase two of the study, when each participant was placed under optimal conditions for them as established in phase one (i.e., internals setting own goals and externals having coach set goals), all four stabilized their on-task behaviours over and above that displayed with the presentation of the alternative treatment.

A final example of an ATD in a sport and exercise setting comes from Sariscsany, Darst and van der Mars (1995) who investigated the effects of three supervision patterns on students' 'on-task' activities (i.e., participants engaging in teacher-directed activities) and practice skill behaviour (i.e., volleyball under-arm and forearm pass). Three experienced PE instructors and three 'off-task' (i.e., inattentive) junior high school males served as participants. The ATD was used to assess on-task behaviour, total practice trials and appropriate practice trials under three supervision patterns. First, close supervision with feedback included a teacher positioned close to the targeted participant providing specific skill feedback for at least 50 per cent of the total practice time. Second, distant supervision with feedback consisted of a teacher being positioned away from the targeted behaviour and issuing specific skill feedback for at least 50 per cent of the practice time. Finally, distant supervision with no feedback entailed the teacher being located away from the target participant for 50 per cent of the practice time and issuing no specific skill feedback. Findings from the study indicated that when the treatments were successfully implemented the percentage of on-task behaviour was significantly higher during active supervision for two target participants (i.e., participants 1 and 2). In contrast, mixed results were demonstrated for total and appropriate practice trials across all three treatments for all participants.

In summary, although the ATD is a flexible, adaptable and well-used design in mainstream applied behavioural research (Barlow et al. 2009), it has received little or no attention from researchers and practitioners in sport and exercise settings (Kinugasa et al. 2004). The challenge of embracing alternative methods such as the ATD to determine treatment or intervention effectiveness exists for those involved in sport and exercise. Finally, although the ATD is the most prevalent single-case method for comparing treatments, variations do exist that extend the flexibility and use of the design in applied behavioural research (Kazdin 1982). The following section introduces the main ATD design variations.

Design variations

The simultaneous-treatment design

A variation to the ATD is the simultaneous-treatment design (STD; Browning 1967; Browning and Stover 1971). In the STD two or more treatments are presented simultaneously in a single case. Typically, the STD evaluates participants' preference among a variety of treatments because they are available at the same time or in the same session. Indeed, the STD allows for the collection of information about treatment preferences (Kazdin 2003; Kazdin and Hartmann 1978; Kratochwill et al. 1984). The STD contrasts with the fast alternation of two or more treatments in the ATD and typically means that participants are not exposed to all treatments equally (Barlow and Hayes 1979). Although the STD has been popular in the single-case literature for a number of decades, only one example exists in applied research (Barlow et al. 2009). In this study Browning (1967) compared the effects of three procedures (praise and attention, verbal admonishment and ignoring) on reducing 'bragging' behaviour (i.e., the telling of untrue and grandiose stories) in a nine-year-old boy. Following a four-week baseline, the practitioners working with the boy (i.e., teams of two therapists) implemented the three procedures simultaneously. The three procedures were balanced across three groups of staff. After each week, the staff members associated with a particular intervention were rotated so that all staff administered all of the interventions to the boy. A unique feature of this study's design was the simultaneous availability of all treatment conditions to the boy. The specific consequence that the boy received for bragging depended on the staff members with whom the boy came into contact. Accordingly, the boy could choose the preferred schedule or treatment as treatments were simultaneously presented; thus he was not equally exposed to each treatment. In fact, the very structure of the STD ensures that the participant will not be equally exposed to all treatments because choice is forced (except in the unlikely event that both treatments are equally preferred; Barlow et al. 2009). The measure of treatment effectiveness was the frequency and duration of bragging incidents over time directed at the various staff members. Data from the participant, presented in Figure 8.9, indicated a preference for verbal admonishment, as indicated by the frequency and duration of bragging, and a lack of preference for ignoring. Therefore, ignoring became the treatment of choice and was continued by all staff.

Despite its unpopularity in applied research, the STD is an important single-case design for understanding individual treatment preferences (Kazdin 2003). In certain applied settings (e.g., when exploring the effectiveness of new

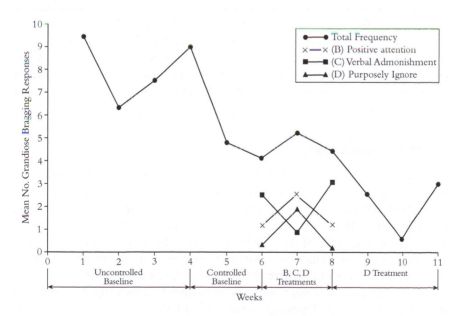

FIGURE 8.9 Total mean frequency of grandiose bragging responses throughout study and for each reinforcement contingency during experimental period. Adapted with permission from R. M. Browning (1967) A same-subject design for simultaneous comparison of three reinforcement contingencies. *Behavior, Research, & Therapy, 5,* 237–243.

interventions) intervention preference may be an important component in understanding both treatment adherence and overall treatment effectiveness. Although exploring intervention preferences is an important facet of applied research, 'preference' is not the same as effectiveness (Barlow et al. 2009). For example, it is possible that participants may choose treatments that are the least invasive and time-consuming and thus possibly less effective in the long term. Despite this obvious limitation, it has been recommended that the STD needs to be implemented in areas of behaviour change where information on treatment preferences is desired (Barlow et al. 2009). Therefore, the STD may be relevant when using techniques that are shrouded in popular misconception or confusion (e.g., hypnosis). To this end, gathering information on why certain techniques were and were not preferred by participants has important implications for applied researchers and practitioners looking to develop and modify innovative modes of intervention (Grindstaff and Fisher 2006). For example, asking a client for feedback about hypnotic procedures allows a practitioner to make modifications to how they deliver the technique in the future. Gathering information on intervention preference is likely to lend itself more closely to qualitative methods (e.g., social validation data) rather than self-report measures. Overall, the STD is a variation of the ATD and typically evaluates participants' preferences among a variety of treatments that are presented simultaneously. Although the STD has been presented as a design useful for determining intervention effectiveness (see Browning 1967; Kazdin 1982), some maintain that the STD is unsuitable for studying differential effects of treatments or conditions and is therefore not well suited to the evaluation of intervention effectiveness (Barlow et al. 2009). To fully understand the appropriateness of the STD in applied settings (e.g., sport and exercise contexts) further research is clearly needed.

Randomization design

The randomization design (Edgington 1966, 1972) in the context of ATDs refers to the presentation of alternative treatments in random order (Barlow et al. 2009; Kazdin 1982). For example, according to Kazdin (1982), baseline (A), treatment 1 (B) and treatment 2 (C) can be presented to participants on a daily basis in the order of A–B–C–B–A–C–A–C–B–C–A–B–C–B–A–B–C–A. Therefore, each day a different condition is presented, on the proviso that each condition is presented an equal number of times. In the intervention phase of an ATD, the alternative interventions must be balanced across stimulus conditions (e.g., time or setting). Therefore, randomly ordering the sequence in which treatments are applied provides researchers with a strategy to organize the presentation of treatments. To illustrate, an exercise psychologist may administer imagery and self-talk on alternative days over a three-week period to evaluate their effects on a client's exercise efficacy. Because the conditions and/or treatments administered on a given day are randomly determined, data are suggested to be more amenable to statistical analysis as a means of determining intervention effectiveness (Edgington 1966, 1972).

In summary, the main design variations related to the ATD are the STD and the randomization design. Although both of these variations have received little application in the applied behavioural literature they are important additions for researchers and practitioners looking for methods to help them derive effective interventions.

Problems and limitations of the alternating-treatments design

As noted previously, the ATD is a flexible and adaptable design but it carries one major limitation: multi-treatment interference (MTI; Campbell and Stanley 1963). In essence, because single-case designs typically involve the repeated measurement of variables from the same participant, data can be *serially dependent* (i.e., data collected at specific moments in time can be influenced by previous measures; see Ottenbacher 1986). This can also occur with data collected under different phases or conditions (Barlow and Hayes 1979). For example, in the ATD, two or more interventions are alternated rapidly over time, making it likely that the effects from one treatment may carry over and influence the following intervention. Therefore, MTI refers to the effect that one treatment has on another; when a participant is exposed to two or more treatments, the experience with one treatment may influence the effectiveness of others (Wolery, Bailey and Sugai 1988). Moreover, MTI is likely to be prevalent in all conditions, including baselines and participants' non-experimental experiences (e.g., participant history; Birnbrauer 1981). When treatments are compared within subjects, four outcomes are possible (Barlow and Hayes 1979): (1) treatments are made *more* effective because of the exposure to other treatment(s), (2) treatments are made *less* effective because of the exposure to other treatment(s), (3) one treatment is made more effective because of the exposure to a first and (4) none of the treatments influences each other. Indeed, the first three potential outcomes lend themselves to the possibility of drawing incorrect or misleading conclusions about intervention effectiveness. Therefore, researchers and practitioners are encouraged to control, detect and describe the presence of MTI within their studies (Barlow et al. 2009; Holcombe et al. 1994). Problems in drawing conclusions about intervention effectiveness also exist in the multi-modal intervention designs seen in the sport and exercise literature (e.g., Barker and Jones 2006; Collins et al. 1999; Freeman et al. 2009; Hanton and Jones 1999; Thelwell and Greenlees 2001). These designs make it difficult to determine which aspect of an intervention has had the greatest effect on target variables.

Continuing with the theme of MTI this section next explores some related concerns (i.e., sequential confounding, carry-over effects and alternation effects; Barlow and Hayes 1979; Kazdin 2003; Ulman and Sulzer-Azaroff 1975) and also explains how MTI can be minimized. First, sequence effects (also known as sequential confounding or order effects) refer to situations in which the order of treatment use influences the potency of one or more of the treatments (Barlow and Hayes 1979). Sequence effects are posited to be particularly acute in single-case designs in which experimental conditions are compared *within* rather than *across* participants, because in nearly all cases participants must experience one treatment before the other; once that experience has occurred it cannot be taken away (Holcombe et al. 1994). For example, a researcher interested in alternating the interventions of pre-performance routines and superstitious behaviours on basketball free-throw shooting may find it difficult to prevent participants from using elements of the pre-performance routine in future shooting conditions. Controlling for sequence effects in ATDs is therefore attempted by rapidly alternating treatment implementation. Using interventions for a brief time is less likely to produce a learning history that could bring about sequence effects (Holcombe et al. 1994). Another recommendation for dealing with sequence effects is to arrange for a random sequencing of treatments within the intervention phase (Barlow et al. 2009).

'Carry-over' effects are influences of one treatment on another that arise from the characteristics of the treatments rather than the order in which they are administered (Holcombe et al. 1994). Carry-over has been suggested to have both positive and negative effects (Barlow and Hayes 1979). *Positive* carry-over effects would be demonstrated if treatment B were more effective when it was alternated with treatment A than if it were the only treatment administered. For example, if a participant is exposed to a relaxation strategy that is alternated with hypnosis it is likely that exposure to relaxation will facilitate the potency of hypnosis given that relaxation is a key aspect common to most hypnotic procedures (Barker and Jones 2006). In contrast, *negative* carry-over would be revealed if treatment B were less effective when it was alternated with treatment A than if it were administered alone. For example, the effectiveness of positive self-talk is likely to be less effective if alternated with thought stopping. Accordingly, from these examples one would make the assumption that treatment A is somehow interfering with the effects that one would see from treatment B if it were delivered alone (Barlow et al. 2009). Because of the potential for sequence effects in ATDs a number of recommendations have been made to limit these effects (Barlow et al. 2009): counterbalancing the order of the treatments, separating treatment sessions with a time interval (e.g., one session per week) and providing slower and discriminable treatment alterations (e.g., Powell and Hake 1971) may all reduce carry-over effects.

This section has identified the major limitations of the ATD – MTI and its associated concerns. Although these limitations of the ATD can be alleviated through the use of the recommendations outlined above, sometimes it may be desirable to assess directly the extent to which MTI and more specifically carry-over effects exist in a study (e.g., McGonigle et al. 1987; Shapiro, Kazdin and McGonigle 1982). Readers are directed to the work of Sidman (1960) for a more detailed account of the procedures involved in assessing MTI.

Evaluation of the design

The ATD has a number of advantages over the reversal and multiple-baseline designs that make it applicable for applied behavioural research (see Barlow et al. 2009; Kazdin 1982). In particular, these advantages make the ATD appropriate for sport and exercise researchers and practitioners (Bryan 1987; Hrycaiko and Martin 1996; Kinugasa et al. 2004). The ATD allows comparison of various treatments and their effects over time, therefore facilitating the literature base on evidence-based practice. Second, it is possible to detect delayed treatment effects because the ATD can involve ongoing baseline as a condition for comparison. Third, the ongoing baseline allows the ATD to be used with variables pertinent to sport and exercise settings (e.g., sport performance, exercise adherence) that occur at unstable rates (McKenzie and Liskevych 1983). Fourth, the concurrent use of treatments in the ATD means that a baseline may not be a requirement or if one is it does not have to be a lengthy baseline, which can be both practically and ethically beneficial (Zhan and Ottenbacher 2001). This is possible because treatments are alternated after short periods of time. Fifth, because of concurrent measurement of treatments, less effective treatments can be detected and terminated easily and without delay (McKenzie and Liskevych 1983). Sixth, the ATD is pertinent to sport and exercise settings because it uses brief samplings of variables rather than lengthy phases as outlined in other single-case designs (e.g., A–B design) and is therefore less intrusive to the training and competition schedules of exercisers and athletes. Finally, the ATD does not involve practitioners having to deal with the ethical dilemma of withdrawing a treatment (e.g., Pates et al. 2001). Overall, the ATD is a strong, flexible and clinically useful strategy for researchers and practitioners engaging in single-case experiments (Barlow et al. 2009).

Summary

The ATD is particularly useful when one wishes to compare two or more potentially effective treatments with each other for the same participant(s). By rapidly alternating treatments it is possible to allow for multiple comparisons of the target variables under each treatment. The major variation to ATD is the STD in which two or more treatments are presented simultaneously, providing information regarding treatment preference of participants. Causal inferences about intervention effectiveness can be difficult in the ATD and STD because of the prevalence of MTI although this apparent threat to internal validity can be reduced by counterbalancing across participants or through the randomization of treatment conditions (Barlow et al. 2009). Overall, the ATD carries many advantages over and above other single-case designs, which make it an attractive approach for applied practitioners and researchers engaged in comparing effective treatments. Finally, the ATD has received a lack of application in sport and exercise in comparison with mainstream applied research.

The previous four chapters have outlined the major tenets of the main design variations (i.e., withdrawal, multiple-baseline, changing-criterion and alternating-treatments designs) pertinent to single-case research methods. Throughout these chapters observations have been made regarding analytical procedures used to determine change or intervention effectiveness. The following chapter provides a more thorough insight into the data analysis procedures involved with single-case data.

Key points

- The alternating-treatments design is a single-case design in which two or more interventions are alternated rapidly in order to compare intervention effectiveness.
- The simultaneous-treatments design is a design variation in which two or more treatments are presented simultaneously in a single case. This design is used to evaluate participants' preference among a variety of treatments.
- Serial dependence is when data are influenced by earlier measures.
- Multi-treatment interference is a threat to the internal validity of an ATD in which the effects of one intervention or treatment interact with other (future) interventions or treatments.
- Sequence effects refers to situations in which the order of treatment or intervention use influences the potency of one or more treatments.
- Carry-over effects are influences of one treatment on another that arise from the characteristics of the treatments rather than the order in which they are administered.
- Counterbalancing is a methodological procedure in an ATD in which the order of treatments is varied (counterbalanced) to eliminate order effects.
- Randomization is a methodological procedure in which the alternating of treatments is not predictable but occurs randomly during the intervention phases.

Guided study

Based upon your reading of Chapter 8 please take some time to respond to the following review questions:

- How does the alternating-treatments design differ from the changing-criterion, withdrawal and multiple-baseline designs?
- Discuss the major tenets of the alternating-treatments design.
- Discuss the major tenets of the simultaneous-treatments design.
- Explain the limitations of the alternating-treatments design.
- Discuss multi-treatment interference and outline (with examples) how its effects can be minimized in the alternating-treatments design.

9

ANALYSING DATA IN SINGLE-CASE RESEARCH

In this chapter, we will:

- outline the experimental process in single-case research;
- explain the advantages and disadvantages of visual analysis of single-case data;
- discuss the use of statistical analysis in single-case research designs.

Introduction

Researchers and practitioners in sport and exercise apply various methods to observe and measure target variables in sport and exercise settings. These methods are necessary for investigators to understand different phenomena valued by athletes, coaches and other professionals in sport and exercise. For instance, a javelin thrower might inquire whether a new technique improves his throwing performance (Collins et al. 1999), a coach might want to know whether self-recording improves attendance at swimming training (McKenzie and Rushall 1974) or a sport psychologist might query whether a hypnosis treatment raises a soccer player's self-efficacy (Barker and Jones 2008). To aid their causes, practitioners need to measure, evaluate and interpret idiographic (i.e., individually focused; see also Chapter 10) or single-case data to ensure that they are meaningful for these clients. If measurement is the guarantee of any science (Mace and Kratochwill 1986), researchers must ensure that they measure what they claim to measure (recall that we addressed how to measure behaviour in Chapter 4). Once the data are collected, the practitioner must analyse them to determine whether a change in the target variable has occurred because of the intervention. Then the researcher or practitioner must interpret and present the data to the appropriate audience –whether it is one's scientific peers or the client with whom one is working.

This chapter is concerned with appropriate types of data analysis for single-case studies. First, we shall examine the experimental process involved in single-case research designs – especially issues concerning the validity and reliability of this research method. Second, we shall explore the traditional method for analysing data in single-case research – visual analysis. Third, we shall present quantitative analysis techniques that researchers and practitioners use to address certain disadvantages of visual analysis. Finally, we shall illustrate how sport and exercise practitioners use various techniques to analyse data in single-case research. Before we begin, however, we introduce a fictitious A–B design (see Figure 9.1) with an aspiring professional golfer that runs alongside this chapter to aid your understanding of data analysis in single-case research.

An amateur golfer approaches you to help her with her golf game. She is twenty-four years old with a scratch handicap and is hoping to become a professional golfer when the golf season ends in six months. She has been performing somewhat erratically in competition and these performances are threatening her imminent career as a professional golfer because she has not had been able to win competitions when she leads the field. After a general consultation with her, and having observed her in competition, you realize that she does not have a clear strategy for playing well under competitive pressure in tournaments. For

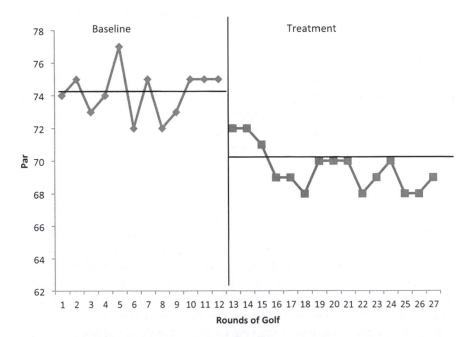

FIGURE 9.1 The golfer's scores per round of golf with horizontal lines indicating the mean scores during baseline and treatment.

March and April you ask her to record the number of shots she required to complete each round of golf. After this baseline stage, when you have collected twelve baseline scores for the dependent (target) variable (number of shots per round of golf), you devise a scoring system to encourage her to self-monitor her use of the 'Smart Golf' approach (Kirschenbaum et al. 1998) to improve and score her mental game in golf. For the next fifteen competitive rounds of golf she self-monitors her progress on the Smart Golf approach and records the number of shots she requires to complete each round of golf. At the end of the treatment phase you have data from a single case that you wish to analyse to determine whether the intervention was successful in lowering her performance scores. We shall consider the options available to you to analyse your data. First, however, we shall explore experimental logic because we want to eliminate alternative hypotheses to explain the outcome of the treatment. To explain, a sound experiment permits the researcher or practitioner to conclude that changes in the target variable emerged because of the treatment and not because of any other factor.

Understanding the experimental process

The goal of experiments in sport and exercise settings, just as in any other experimental research, is to understand the causal relations among independent and dependent variables (see also Chapters 1 and 2). In single-case research designs, researchers manipulate a particular treatment (independent variable) and examine its effect on the target variable (dependent variable). We can measure changes in the target variable to understand what determines this change. If the study is methodologically sound, we can conclude that the changes in the target variable emerged from the treatment or independent variable rather than as a result of any other factor (Morgan and Morgan 2009). In our example above, we might conclude that changes in the performance scores of the golfer were due to the self-monitoring intervention rather than any other factor. When we make this assumption, we refer to the 'internal validity' of the experiment. The internal validity or 'experimental realism' of an experiment represents the degree to which the researcher is confident that the changes in the dependent variable emerged because of changes in the independent variable rather than because of any other factor (Aronson, Ellsworth, Carlsmith and Gonzales 1990). To be confident of this change, the researcher carefully designs each experiment. For example, Smith, Smoll and Barnett (1995) conducted a field experiment in baseball to assess the usefulness of a social support and stress reduction programme for factors affecting performance anxiety in child athletes. Using a group design, coaches in the experimental condition received pre-season training on behavioural guidelines to reduce anxiety. The no-treatment control group did not receive the coach training. After the experiment, compared with the no-treatment control group, interviews with the children trained by coaches in the experimental group revealed that they evaluated their coaches more positively and had more fun and that the teams had a higher level of attraction among players regardless of the 'won–lost' records. As long as group differences in these factors were not attributable to any other cause, the most plausible explanation for this difference would be that they were due to the independent variable – namely coach training. This assumption also applies to single-case research designs.

What is 'validity'?

'Validity' is the degree to which a measuring instrument measures what it purports to measure (Nunnally and Bernstein 1994). Three types of validity have been identified in psychometric research: construct validity, predictive validity and content validity (Gliner, Morgan and Leech 2009). Construct validity is the degree to which a measuring instrument assesses the psychological construct that it purports to measure. Predictive validity refers to the extent to which a measuring instrument predicts some criterion index of the construct in question. Finally, content validity is the degree to which a measuring instrument reflects a clearly defined content area (Primavera, Allison and Alfonso 1996). In other words, does the content that constitutes the measure represent the concept one is trying to measure? (Gliner et al. 2009) In practice, a valid measure will have a distinct purpose and we must ensure that a measure we choose is a valid instrument for our purpose. For example, a sphygmomanometer measures blood pressure excellently but heart rate poorly. In single-case research, we are often engaged with direct sampling of behaviour. We might expect that there is little interference from the observer but on closer inspection, as we recall from Chapters 3 and 4, certain characteristics of human behaviour may interfere with the measurement process. Without a clear, objective definition of the target variable, it would be difficult to collect accurate, reliable data about that behaviour. For example, Smith and Ward (2006) conducted a behavioural intervention to improve performance in collegiate American football. They measured the percentage of correct blocks used to determine whether the wide receiver blocked effectively. To ensure that the observer recorded a block correctly, the authors defined a correct block precisely in behavioural terms and an independent observer recorded each player's performance to determine the reliability of the observational data.

Internal validity

The causal attribution logic of single-case research designs resembles that of group designs; however, the data collection and analysis strategies differ between these research methods. Using single-case designs, we observe, measure and record the target variable under baseline and treatment conditions (Cooper et al. 2007). When we compare the two conditions, we draw conclusions about the effects of the independent variable. Briefly, what we are aiming to do is eliminate alternative explanations for behaviour change. In other words, we want to be certain that we can account for any changes detected in the dependent variable simply as a function of the manipulation of the independent variable only. So, could other variables account for the changes in the dependent variable? And if so, what are these variables? Because many threats to the internal validity of an experiment exist, we must be aware of them and assess their influence on our design. To begin with, a variable might confound the results of our experiment. For instance, if the aspiring professional golfer we introduced at the beginning of this chapter improved her golf performance following a treatment using a self-monitoring strategy, we might conclude that the changes were due to that treatment. If, however, she had changed *coaches* during the treatment phase and her new coach taught her a better putting technique that reduced her number of putts per round of golf, we, as researchers and practitioners, would be less confident that this golfer's better performance emerged because of the treatment alone. In this example, the new putting technique taught by the coach represents a confounding variable because it makes less certain any conclusions about the manipulated independent variable.

Other threats to the internal validity of a study include factors such as history, maturation and regression towards the mean (Campbell and Stanley 1963). The history effect refers to the fact that, sometimes, certain variables outside the experimenter's environment that are not controlled by the experimenter influence the dependent variable. If, for example, a basketball coach was teaching children to react assertively in basketball training but these children were also receiving lessons from their teacher at school about assertiveness, then any conclusions about the effects of the basketball coach's programme would not be strong because of this history variable at school. The maturation effect implies that changes in the dependent variable over time emerge because of normal developmental (also know as maturational) factors, rather than as a result of the manipulated independent variable. This threat is possible in studies of infants or young children because, if a researcher conducts a study over one year, for instance, we might attribute any changes to young children just 'getting older' rather than to the programme we had implemented (Morgan and Morgan 2009). Finally, regression towards the mean is the statistical tendency for a data series to gravitate towards the centre of a distribution (see Chapter 3). Put simply, if people are tested repeatedly, those who score below average the first time will probably do better the next time – and those who score above average the first time will probably do worse the next time. Another example of such regression is that children of very tall parents tend to be taller than average children, but shorter than the average of the parents' heights. If a boxer presents extreme scores on an anxiety scale, we might expect these scores to decrease over time, regardless of whether he receives any therapy to treat his anxiety. Researchers may accidentally appraise change in the dependent variable from the manipulated independent variable.

Other biases arise in research, such as sampling, participant and experimenter effects, which affect the conclusions we draw from our research. Certain 'nuisance variables' affect our research process because, although such variables bear no specific interest for the researcher (e.g., personality traits, social class), they might explain the existence or absence of group differences at the end of the experiment (Kazdin 2003). When we come across an athlete, we study that athlete without much regard for his or her representativeness, even as a athlete. Participant effects can cause a participant's behaviour to be an artefact of the experiment rather than a natural response to a manipulation. As outlined in Chapter 3, features of an experiment that appear to demand a particular response are demand characteristics (Orne 1962). If participants uncover the hypothesis, it might influence compliant participants to react to confirm the hypothesis. If the participants worry about evaluation, it might cause them to act unnaturally. We refer to this phenomenon as evaluation apprehension (Rosenberg 1969). Experimenter effects occur when the experimenter is aware of the hypothesis and inadvertently gives cues causing the participants to behave in ways that confirm the hypothesis. In social psychology, for example, psychology undergraduates have typically been the research participants in many laboratory experiments (Sears 1986) because they are readily available. Unfortunately, such reliance on psychology undergraduates may appear to have distorted our view of social behaviour – but experimental social psychologists argue that *theories*, not experimental findings, are generalized (Hogg and Vaughan 2008). In any case, most single-case research designs in sport and exercise involve sport performers and exercisers from the broad spectrum of this population.

With all these threats to internal validity, how can we be sure that we draw legitimate conclusions about our study? Group and single-case research designs can overcome these challenges by two processes: replication and repeated measurement of the dependent variable (Campbell and Stanley 1963). Replication allows us to draw comparisons between the participant's behaviour during the baseline and treatment phases of the study. For example, single-case researchers typically introduce the independent variables at various times across behaviours, participants or settings in multiple-baseline designs (Barlow and Hersen 1984). Based on the requirements of a given design (e.g., A–B–A) we would expect that each phase change is an opportunity to observe changes in the target variable. It is improbable that each phase change would coincide with a confounding variable, and more replications means that the likelihood of a coincidental confounding variable decreases with each phase change (Morgan and Morgan 2009). Cyclical patterns such as sleep or hormonal fluctuations can influence human behaviour, and such systematic, recurring patterns in the target variable that are not the direct result of the treatment variable are known as cyclic variation or cyclicity. If there are identical fluctuations in trends, such cyclicity makes estimating treatment effects problematic. To counter this effect, researchers should consider all possible sources of variation a priori and measure their occurrence (e.g., hormonal changes) as well as extending the phase lengths (Barlow et al. 2009). A second method to increase the internal validity of single-case designs is through repeated measures. Because we are constantly monitoring the relevant target variable, we can control many threats to the internal validity of our experiment. For example, we take multiple measures of the target variable in the baseline before introducing the treatment where statistical regression should be evident. If no change in the baseline scores emerges, then we can be confident that statistical regression is unlikely to be a threat to internal validity. Repeated measurement also counteracts the threat of maturation because we would expect developmental changes to occur during baseline measures as well as during treatment (Morgan and Morgan 2009).

External validity

In general, the term 'external validity' or 'mundane realism' refers to the similarity between the conditions encountered by participants in a given study and those pertaining in the real world (Aronson et al. 1990). In single-case research, external validity refers to the extent to which an effect that is documented in one study has relevance for people and behaviours in other settings. We value the external validity of interventions in sport and exercise because we want to show whether the intervention is valuable for other sport performers or exercisers in similar contexts. But cultural, historical and age group limits are present in many studies and it will not be practical to account for all these factors. For our results to be truly generalizable, we should ensure participant representativeness alongside the representativeness of settings and manipulations (Deese 1972; Mook 1983); however, this is not always possible or desirable. In short, we are not just making generalizations; we are *testing* them (Mook 1983). In the laboratory, our aim for collecting data may be to 'predict real-life behaviour in the real world' (Mook 1983, p. 114). If this is so, then the hurdle of external validity confronts us; when it is not our aim, external validity is trivial. Laboratory and field research unfolds to develop theories and practical applications for sport and exercise. But researchers must control their experiments carefully because, without such care, unverifiable explanations will emerge. Thomas (1980, p. 267) shared a humorous anecdote about such research and inductive reasoning:

> A researcher spends several weeks training a cockroach to jump. The bug became well trained and would leap high in the air on the command 'Jump'. The researcher then began to manipulate his independent variable, which was to remove the bug's legs one at a time. Upon removing the first leg, the researcher said, 'Jump' and the bug did. He then removed the second, third, fourth, and fifth leg and said 'Jump' after each leg was removed, and the bug jumped every time. Upon removing the sixth leg and giving the 'Jump' command, the bug just lay there. The researcher's conclusion from this research was: 'When all the legs are removed from a cockroach, the bug becomes deaf'!

Making sense of the data

Rainer Martens (1987, p. 53) endorsed the value of applied research by suggesting that 'sport psychologists can acquire knowledge much more rapidly by developing solutions to practical problems'. Whether or not we accept this argument, it is clear that in professional practice we need to evaluate our treatments to save time and resources as well as to establish our accountability (Anderson et al. 2002; Bryan 1987). These goals place the onus on sport psychologists (and sport and exercise scientists) to ensure that they avoid ineffective intervention strategies but also understand which elements of a given intervention package work best for individual effectiveness. As we have repeatedly emphasized in this book, single-case research designs are preferable to group designs in sport settings when dealing with small populations such as elite, injured or overtrained athletes because recruiting a sufficiently large sample to detect a practically significant effect is costly and often impractical (Kinugasa et al. 2004). As the field of applied sport and exercise psychology grows, the demand for accountability and credibility increases (Bryan 1987; Hemmings and Holder 2009; Smith 1989). Therefore, sport and exercise psychologists require methods to analyse the data they collect about their client(s). Data analysis procedures in single-case research in sport and exercise typically follow two routes: a graphical approach and/or a quantitative approach. The graphical approach presents data graphically, for example an observer assesses the target variable over time (see Figure 9.1). We can display data simply without much reorganization. The quantitative or inferential statistical analysis approach often follows the graphical approach, which is typical in behavioural research (Johnston and Pennypacker 1993). More recently, researchers and practitioners have included quantitative approaches to address certain drawbacks in the graphical approach. We shall present these two approaches in the following sections.

The graphical approach

Although many methods exist to analyse single-case data, the traditionally favoured approach used by practitioners in sport and exercise contexts is visual analysis. Visual analysis offers a basic method to analyse single-case research data and comprises visually inspecting data and judging whether a treatment has produced a significant change in the dependent variable (Bloom et al. 2009; Kinugasa et al. 2004). In Figure 9.1, just as in Chapters 5–8, the pictorial illustration of the data makes this system of data analysis manageable and self-explanatory. Although this system seems to allow us to interpret behaviour change easily, we shall explain later that unless we use specific rules to understand changes in the data we can draw inaccurate inferences about the data. For instance, even experienced reviewers of behavioural journals looking at the same data disagree on what they see or draw different conclusions from time to time (DeProspero and Cohen 1979). One way to support visual analysis of single-case data is to use statistical analysis; however, statistical analysis also has some drawbacks for researchers and practitioners, which we will discuss later.

Displaying the data

Graphed data are usually presented with a measure of time on the abscissa (the horizontal axis) and the dependent variable on the ordinate (the vertical axis). As was seen in Chapters 5–8, the independent variable contains two or more levels of treatment separated by two or more blocks of time. Three interpretative principles are used for the graphic analysis of single-case data: central location, variability and trend. Many graphic displays in sport and exercise research present single observations as data points so differences in data level between and within treatment phases reveal treatment effectiveness (Franklin, Gorman, Beasley and Allison 1996). When data are plotted individually, 'level' represents central location. Level can represent mean, median or mode. In Figure 9.1 we presented level using mean scores. Variability refers to deviations above and below level (or mean scores in Figure 9.1). We can display this variability using range bars (Parsonson and Baer 1978) and range lines. Finally, trend comprises lines drawn on a graph that offer the best linear fit of the data and demonstrate how the data change over time.

Central tendency refers to measures of the location of the middle of a distribution. The mean is the most common measure of central tendency but researchers also use median (i.e., the value that is in the middle of all the values) and mode (i.e., the most frequently occurring value among all the values). The mean refers to the average among all the scores; it is the sum of a set of values, divided by the number of values. The median proves useful because outliers (i.e., extreme scores) do not influence it; however, it does not consider the numerical value of every score as the mean does. In that sense, extreme scores (i.e., outliers) affect the mean, dragging the mean towards the outlier (Bloom et al. 2009). One way to overcome this distortion is to use a trimmed mean (Rosenthal and Rosnow 2007). We can calculate a trimmed mean by excluding a certain percentage (e.g., 10 per cent) of the highest and lowest values and then calculating the mean from the remaining scores. Similar to medians, trimmed means protect against distortions created by outliers but they also make greater use of the information available in a set of data.

To understand a set of scores, not only do we need measures of central tendency but also measures of variation. A measure of variation refers to the degree to which data deviate from the overall pattern of data (Bloom et al. 2009). Researchers normally use the range and standard deviation. The range represents the difference between the highest and the lowest value in a set of scores. The value of the range depends on the extreme values in a set of scores. In other words, if the extreme scores are uncharacteristic of most scores, then the range cannot provide an accurate reflection of the variation in a set of scores. Similar to means scores, a trimmed range can help deal with outliers (Rosenthal and

Rosnow 1991). Again, a trimmed range is calculated when a certain percentage of the highest and lowest values are excluded. One commonly used trimmed range is the interquartile range. We calculate the interquartile range by finding the scores that are at the twenty-fifth percentile and the seventy-fifth percentile and noting their difference (Clark-Carter 2009). The range and trimmed range allow us to see changes in variability from one phase to another.

The standard deviation, unlike the median, range and trimmed range, accounts for all numerical values in a set of scores. It tells us how much a score in a given distribution of scores varies from the mean. Standard deviation is the preferred measure of spread when analysing data because it is a measure of spread that relates to the mean. We express standard deviation units in the same units as the original measure (Clark-Carter 2009).

Measures of trend

If we rely on the mean or median to summarize the data for a golfer's emotional experience over time, we might be misled by what we see. When the target variable is increasing or decreasing systematically over time, we suggest that there is a trend in the data. If we map a line onto the data, we can summarize a trend – we call this a trend line. The greater the incline or decline, the greater the change over time. And the greater the incline (i.e., steepness of the slope), the greater the change in the target variable. The slope tells us the average amount of change from one time point to the next. A trend line can be constructed by drawing a line that best represents the trend of scores. Drawing this line, however, challenges most researchers because the data rarely fall along a straight line. In this instance, we usually eyeball the data and draw a line accordingly; however, this method lacks accuracy, prompting researchers to construct a line that best summarizes the trend in a target variable. Researchers call this line a 'celeration line'. A celeration line forms from the root of the terms 'acceleration' and 'deceleration' (Morgan and Morgan 2009). This line connects the midpoints of the first and second halves of a phase. With these lines we can describe the effectiveness of the intervention. We can construct a celeration line for the baseline and intervention phase. Then we can see the differences between two phases clearly. Another method is to extend the celeration line from the baseline construction through the intervention period (Bloom et al. 2009). With this line it is possible to predict the trend in the intervention phase based on the baseline phase and observe any deviations from this line that result from the intervention.

We present two methods to superimpose trend lines on the graphed data: the least-squares regression and split-middle methods. The least-squares regression method minimizes the squared vertical distances between data points by calculating a regression line from the slope and intercept (Franklin, Allison and Gorman 1996; Jaccard and Becker 1990). Spreadsheets such as Microsoft Excel contain a function to calculate least-squares regression lines. The regression line is presented as follows:

$$Y = a + bX$$

where the slope is represented by:

$$b_1 = \frac{\Sigma (x-\bar{x}) \times (y-\bar{y})}{\Sigma (x-\bar{x})^2}$$

and the intercept is calculated as:

$$b_0 = y - (b_1 \times X)$$

Using the split-middle technique (White 1971) and a binomial test offers a non-parametric method to reveal the nature of trend in data (Kinugasa et al. 2004). Once the trend lines are determined, we can use a binomial test to determine the statistical significance of the treatment effect. The split-middle method can be calculated as follows (Franklin et al. 1996, p. 129):

1 Divide the time-series plot into halves along the abscissa (horizontal axis).
2 Locate the median time value and median of the dependent variable for each time-series half. When the number of data points in a time series is uneven, the middle points can be randomly assigned to either half or assigned to each half with the line being fitted twice.
3 Make a coordinate from the intersection of the time and dependent variable medians and extend a line through the coordinates of each half.

Marlow, Bull, Heath and Shambrook (1998) used the split-middle technique to analyse the effect of a pre-performance routine on the water polo penalty shot among three experienced male water polo players. Although mean performance scores increased for all three players between pre- and post-intervention phases, a split-middle technique described performance trends and changes further.

Understanding changes in level and trend

As we have explained in this book, one of the major advantages of single-case research designs is that they allow a researcher or practitioner to examine the *continuous measurement* of the target variable. In short, they enable investigators to detect any changes in the target variable over time. For example, Figure 9.2 illustrates the number of minutes a cyclist devotes to riding his bicycle during the pre-season. For the past few seasons, this cyclist did not spend enough time

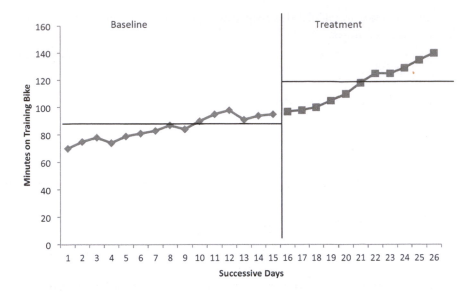

FIGURE 9.2 The cyclist's time spent on his training bike with the horizontal lines representing mean scores during baseline and treatment.

building his endurance during the pre-season and his performances suffered later in the season. We can see that the number of minutes spent cycling in the pre-season increases steadily throughout the baseline and treatment phases. The increasing trend through the baseline and treatment phases suggests that something other than the intervention might be responsible for this trend. During the baseline, for example, the number of minutes spent cycling increased from day 1 to day 15; therefore, there might be a reason to believe that the intervention was not effective. Researchers and practitioners aim for a stable baseline with no obvious upwards or downwards trend (Morgan and Morgan 2009). Treatments are difficult to interpret when the trend in the baseline is in a direction intended by the treatment. But these are the challenges that most practitioners encounter in applied practice, and waiting until the baseline stabilizes often contravenes the needs of the client. The length of a baseline depends on at least two criteria: stability and time. Stability refers to an apparently unchanging baseline – one that does not contain unpredictable cycles or broad fluctuations. The baseline should help you to gauge what might happen to the target variable in the future. However, it may not be either realistic or ethical to adhere strictly to these criteria.

Understanding changes in variability

Researchers often examine the baseline and treatment phases of an intervention to determine whether variability is consistent in each phase. One goal for a sport and exercise practitioner might be to reduce the variability of the target variable during the treatment phase. For example, a client might run four times per week but the number of minutes that the client runs fluctuates excessively, reducing the training effect. In Figure 9.3, the client's runs vary between fifty minutes and twenty-five minutes.

The goal of the behaviour change programme might be to help the client to run with increasing intensity for between thirty-five and forty minutes using a self-management strategy. The treatment phases indicate that the client's runs now vary between thirty-five and forty minutes without any change in the frequency of runs. The variability exhibited during the baseline phase is reduced in the treatment phase.

Determining behaviour change using visual analysis

How do we know if a treatment (intervention programme) has had an effect on a dependent variable in single-case research? Hrycaiko and Martin (1996) outlined five commonly used guidelines to determine the efficacy of a treatment on the target variable. First, the final few data points in the baseline should be reasonably stable, or in a direction *opposite* to that predicted by the effects of the treatment. Second, the more times that an effect is replicated, the greater our confidence can be that an effect has been observed. Third, few overlapping data points between adjacent baseline and treatment phases also enhances our confidence that we have observed a legitimate effect. Fourth, the sooner the

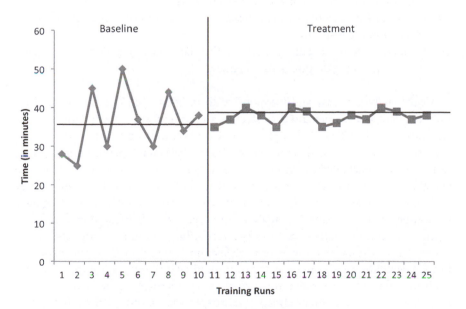

FIGURE 9.3 The runner's time spent on training runs with the horizontal lines representing mean scores during baseline and treatment.

effect is observed, the greater our confidence that an effect has been observed. Finally, if the effect is large we are most confident that a change has occurred. But the size of effect relates to scientific assessment and clinical assessment. With scientific assessment we are interested in the level of performance in the intervention compared with that in the baseline, but in clinical assessment we are interested in aspects of social validity. Parsonson and Baer (1978, pp. 120–130) offer a more detailed heuristic to guide analysis of graphed data. These guidelines include:

1 Stability of baseline: Baselines should be stable and not drift towards improvement.
2 Variability within phases: If phases demonstrate increased variability, more data are needed.
3 Variability between phases: When relatively stable treatment phase data follow variable data, a degree of experimental control is apparent.
4 Overlap between scores of adjacent phases: The less overlap, the greater the treatment effect.
5 Number of data points in each phase: More data points is better, especially with variability, overlap or drift in the data.
6 Changes in trend within phases: Collect more data if trends appear unclear.
7 Changes in trend between adjacent phases: Strong treatment effects are inferred from dramatic changes between adjacent phases.
8 Changes in level between phases: Strong treatment effects are inferred from dramatic changes between adjacent phases.
9 Analysis of data across similar phases: A treatment effect is inferred when replication is consistent.
10 Evaluation of the overall pattern of the data: The overall pattern might prove convincing despite isolated faults.

Visual analysis is easy and inexpensive to use – it produces graphs to simplify the data and understand the effect of a treatment on a dependent variable (Kinugasa et al. 2004). Although single-case research emphasizes the visual analysis of data in graphs (Parsonson and Baer 1986) and depends upon replication to make reliable causal inferences (Sidman 1960), some critics argue that visual analysis is limited as a research tool to detect whether treatment effects are present or absent. Some researchers debate whether visually inspecting data should be the only method to analyse single-case data because they recognize weaknesses in this data analysis strategy. According to these researchers, visual inspection is a subjective mode of analysis and is therefore prone to biases of human perception and contaminated by individual differences. Subjective visual analysis offers the researcher no formal or standardized criteria for making judgements about treatment effects (DeProspero and Cohen 1979; Wolery and

Harris 1982). Therefore, despite the guidelines, some researchers argue that visual inspection is susceptible to idiosyncratic interpretation and therefore to error (Furlong and Wampold 1981, 1982; Ottenbacher 1990; Ottenbacher and Cusick 1991). Supporting this idea, DeProspero and Cohen (1979) found that research participants presented with graphed single-case data disagreed about the presence or absence of treatment effects. But disagreement among those judging the presence or absence of treatment effects is also apparent even among trained professionals. Harbst, Ottenbacher and Harris (1991) examined the inter-rater reliability of physical and occupational therapists to make visual judgements from graphed data from A–B (baseline–treatment) designs. Low inter-rater agreement emerged for the sample suggesting that interpreting data across raters may be inconsistent or conflicting. Probing this problem further, it seems that disagreements in judgements about single-case data are typically related to particular characteristics of the data such as amount of trend or magnitude of effect (Bailey 1984; Ottenbacher 1990) and the amount of serial dependency or autocorrelation in the data (Bengali and Ottenbacher 1998). To enhance the veracity of single-case methods, many data-analytic strategies have emerged that we will explore later.

When using statistical techniques to conclude that the treatment has had an effect on the target variable, the effect has to be statistically significant; however, small changes in some variables might be useful to some clients. In single-case designs, similar to group designs, small effects can be impressive. Small effects might have major implications in a practical context, accumulate in ongoing processes over time to large effects and may be important theoretically (Abelson 1985; Prentice and Miller 1992). Prentice and Miller (1992) explained that the size of an effect depends not only on the relationship between the independent and dependent variables but also on the operations used to generate the data. Many examples from psychology support such claims. If, for example, an elite sprinter improves his running performance time by 5 per cent, that sprinter might move to the top of the world rankings. In sport settings, small but reliable changes are often critical to the performance of a sport performer so practitioners must recognize the context in which the change has occurred and the significance of change for the performer. Because behavioural analysis is concerned with clinical as much as statistical significance, when practitioners work with clients they must ask at least two questions (Bailey and Birch 2002): First, is there a cause–effect relationship between the independent and dependent variable? And if so, is it of sufficient size to interest anyone? The difficulty in making a conclusion about graphic data is the amount of variability and trending. If there is too much variability in either the baseline or the treatment conditions, it may be difficult to tell if there was a cause and effect relationship. If there is any significant trending during the baseline or intervention, it is difficult to tell if you had an effect.

The percentage of non-overlapping data statistic

A simple and useful method for analysing single-case data is the percentage of non-overlapping data (PND) statistic (Scruggs and Mastropieri 2001; Scruggs, Mastropieri, Cook and Escobar 1986). The PND statistic is calculated by recording the percentage of treatment data that overlap with the most 'extreme' data point in the baseline (Morgan and Morgan 2009). In the example in Figure 9.4, inappropriate on-court behaviours in tennis are presented across baseline and treatment phases. The data point in training session seven of the baseline is used to draw the horizontal line that extends into the treatment phase. During training session seven, Andy displayed fifteen instances of inappropriate behaviour. In this example, the PND represents the number of data points in the treatment phase that do not overlap with the value fifteen. Seven of the ten data points in the treatment phase of the graph have a value less than fifteen; therefore the PND is 70 per cent. Researchers often report this statistic in single-case research because it is easy to calculate and interpret; however, its value to quantify an intervention's effectiveness is limited for a few reasons (Morgan and Morgan 2009). First, White (1987) argued that the PND is not sensitive to data with baseline trends; for example it does not detect if the non-overlapping data points are all at the end of the treatment phase suggesting that perhaps the intervention did have an effect eventually. In addition, using a

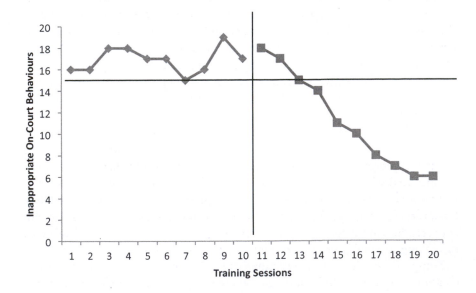

FIGURE 9.4 The tennis player's inappropriate on-court behaviours with a horizontal line drawn through the most extreme low point in the baseline and extended into the treatment phase.

single value may not accurately represent large data sets (Parker, Hagan-Burke and Vannest 2007).

Measures of effect size

To compare phases of a study (e.g., baseline with intervention) or to compare the results of different studies it is possible to use 'effect size' statistics. Effect sizes allow us to compare the results of studies independently of sample size. Although measures of central tendency, variation and trend are valuable, effect size is more precise. Effect sizes quantify the amount of change between phases allowing researchers to compare how effective interventions are across phases or different single-system designs (Bloom et al. 2009). We introduce two methods to calculate effect size: Δ-index and g-index.

Δ-Index

This method of calculating effect size uses the following formula:

$$ES = \frac{M_B - M_A}{SD_A}$$

In this formula, we subtract the mean of all scores in the baseline period (M_A) from the mean of all scores in the intervention period (M_B). We divide this figure by the standard deviation of the scores in the baseline period (SD_A). The basic Δ-index tells us how different the scores in the intervention phase are from the scores in the baseline phase. Cohen (1988) suggested a rough guide to interpret effect size. Cohen considered a value of 0.20 as small, 0.50 as medium and 0.80 as large. This interpretation, however, emerged from group data rather than from single-system data. To address this fact, Parker and Vannest (2009) examined 200 single-system design A–B contrasts and suggested a more appropriate interpretation of effect size for single-system data: small effect size < 0.87; medium effect size 0.87–2.67; and large effect size > 2.67.

g-Index

Using the Δ effect size is not always appropriate, especially when there is a trend in the data. In such cases it is possible to use a g-index. A g-index is computed using the formula

$$P_B - P_A$$

where P_B is the proportion of the intervention scores in the desired zone of the extended baseline trend and P_A is the proportion of baseline scores in the desired zone of the baseline trend line.

Evaluating change using tests of statistical significance

Visual analysis of data has several strengths but also certain limitations – perhaps most importantly its subjectivity; however, we can overcome that challenge and present more objective interpretations of our data using other methods such as quantitative statistics. Statistical tests to analyse single-system data are abundant (e.g., Ferron 2002; Huitema 2004; Parker and Brossart 2003) and we highlight some in the coming paragraphs that are readily available to researchers and practitioners. These tests can help you to decide whether or not change occurred from one phase to the next. We shall discuss two statistical tests, chi-square (χ^2) test and t-test, but first we shall explain what assumptions we must make before we can use these tests validly.

Parametric tests make certain assumptions about the nature of certain parameters for the measures that have been taken and their calculation involves estimation from the sample data of population parameters (Clark-Carter 2009; Gliner et al. 2009). One assumption is that the population of scores from which the data came is normally distributed. No person should contribute more than one score and no person should influence another's score. If the criteria for a parametric test are not fulfilled, then using that parametric test is inappropriate. In this case, a non-parametric test might be appropriate. Although some researchers mistakenly believe that non-parametric tests are free of any assumptions about the distribution of the data, this is not true (Clark-Carter 2009). Non-parametric tests require certain assumptions about the data to be fulfilled. For example, the chi-square statistic (which is a non-parametric statistic) assumes that data are *independent*. In other words, each measurement of a variable is unaffected by other measures of that variable. In group designs, this assumption is usually met because measuring a variable in one participant is usually independent from measuring that variable in another participant (Morgan and Morgan 2009). Unfortunately, in single-case research, all measures of the target variable come from the same participant over time. Because behaviour is a continuous phenomenon showing serial dependency, we expect this occurrence in single-case data. We refer to serial dependency as 'autocorrelation', which presents problems for traditional significance tests (Gottman 1981; Gottman and Rushe 1994; Matyas and Greenwood 1991).

Time-series analysis

Researchers and practitioners apply time-series analysis to determine the nature, direction and magnitude of the relationship between variables measured over time. Time-series analysis is beneficial because it does not depend on stable baselines yet it can establish performance changes between adjacent phases (Kinugasa et al. 2004). Statistically significant changes in slope and level can be calculated between phases. Slope denotes the degree of the angle of a linear line and this value represents the rate of change from one phase to the next. Level denotes the magnitude of change in data when the treatment was introduced.

When practitioners analyse short time-series data, they must overcome specific challenges because visual inference is unreliable with such data and many statistical procedures cannot control type I error (i.e., an erroneous inference of a statistically significant difference between phases) because positive autocorrelation is underestimated (Crosbie 1993). Crosbie (1993) developed an interrupted time-series analysis procedure (ITSACORR) to estimate autocorrelation more accurately with acceptable power. ITSACORR assumes that data are autocorrelated and each phase (e.g., baseline, treatment) has a different intercept and slope. The amount of autocorrelation is estimated using an algebraic manipulation and this parameter is used to control for autocorrelation when using general linear modelling. General linear modelling determines whether the change from baseline to treatment and the difference between the two intercepts and between the two slopes are statistically significant (Callow and Waters 2005; Crosbie 1995). An omnibus F-value demonstrates the change from baseline phase to treatment phase; a t-value for the intercept demonstrates whether the dependent variable has increased or decreased from the final data point in the baseline phase to the first data point in the treatment phase; and a t-value for the slope demonstrates changes in the trend of the data (Callow and Waters 2005). More elaborate details on the assumptions and procedure of ITSACORR are presented in Crosbie (1995). Callow and Waters (2005) examined the effect of kinaesthetic imagery on the sport confidence of three flat-race horse jockeys. They used ITSACORR to analyse the sport confidence data, indicating that two of the three jockeys significantly increased their sport confidence.

Crosbie (1993) recommended that each phase should contain between ten and twenty scores to accurately estimate autocorrelation and power; however, he claims that ITSACORR can maintain an acceptable level of type I and II error with five data points in each phase. For best practice, however, at least ten data points are recommended for the baseline and treatment phases (Callow and Waters 2005). The extent of autocorrelation in single-case research remains dubious (Houle 2009). Some researchers have developed methods of analysing time-series data containing autocorrelation but again the validity of these methods remains problematic (Huitema 2004; Huitema and McKean 2000).

We use a chi-square test to examine whether a statistically significant difference emerges between the expected and observed frequencies in different categories. First, however, we must determine frequencies and we can do that using a celeration line that we described earlier in this chapter. If we want the target variable to increase then we consider the area above the celeration line as the positive zone, but if we want the target variable to decrease then we consider the area below the celeration line as the positive zone (Bloom et al. 2009). Chi-square hypothesizes that the differences between expected and observed frequencies of baseline and intervention periods will be statistically significant. It assumes that data are independent and each cell in a chi-square test should have an adequate sample of at least five. This technique is relatively new with single-system designs and requires greater assessment to determine its value for practitioners.

Another method to determine change between stages in single-systems data is the t-test. Although a researcher can determine whether a statistically significant difference between the mean score in one phase and the mean score in another phase exists, a t-test requires particular parametric assumptions about the data. For example, we should not use a t-test when the data are autocorrelated, unless we transform the data to remove autocorrelation (Kenny and Judd 1986). When a trend in the data emerges, the mean ceases to accurately summarize the data; yet many single-system data sets have a visually noticeable trend in one or both phases (Parker, Cryer and Byrns 2006).

We mentioned earlier that we must fulfil certain assumptions about the data before we can validly use a parametric test. However, in a study of 166 published A–B contrasts, 67 per cent had unacceptable autocorrelation, 51 per cent violated the normality assumption and 45 per cent of the data sets violated the equality of variance assumption (Parker and Hagan-Burke 2007). In group designs, researchers approximate sample sizes to generate a statistically significant difference between groups. In single-case designs, the larger the number of data points per phase, the greater the likelihood of detecting an existing difference between phases (Bloom et al. 2009). And the larger the number of data points, the smaller the difference it is possible to detect. Bloom et al. (2009) recommended having at least six observations per phase, giving a reasonable chance of detecting a large effect size (i.e., $\Delta = 1.50$). For a small effect size, at least thirteen observations per phase are required (Orme 1991).

Revusky's R_n (test of ranks)

One statistical test that has been proposed to examine the effect of an intervention in multiple-baseline designs is the R_n, test of ranks (Revusky 1967). In multiple-baseline designs, data are collected across several outcomes, settings or participants and the treatment effect is assessed based on the performance of each of the baselines at the point when the treatment was introduced (Kinugasa et al. 2004). In a multiple-baseline design, the performance of all participants, for example, would be ranked for that point in time when the treatment is introduced. Ranks are based on the percentage change in level from baseline to the time when the treatment is introduced to any of the participants. The R_n statistic is calculated by summing the ranks across all participants each time the treatment is introduced. Unfortunately, this test is also susceptible to the effects of autocorrelation (Sierra, Quera and Solanas 2000).

Summary

Effective, efficient and useful data analysis techniques are invaluable in single-case research designs in sport and exercise. Sport and exercise practitioners encounter many challenges in research and professional practice in providing a service that meets the needs of the client. Often group designs are neither functional nor practical in sport psychology (Zaichkowsky 1980). For example, there is the ethical issue of having a no-treatment control group, which would be unacceptable to many coaches and athletes. If a researcher compared two intervention strategies it would be possible to eliminate the no-treatment control group; however, finding enough athletes with the same problem is complex. Group designs, although valuable, may misrepresent the individual. In psychotherapy techniques, some individuals might improve and others get worse, presenting a group average showing no effect of treatment. This can also happen in sport. Group designs typically use statistical analysis to determine the probability that the differences between groups were due to change (Bryan 1987). When within-group variability is low, small but significant differences between groups may emerge, but when within-group variability is high, small changes may not achieve statistical significance, perhaps doing injustice to a useful intervention. Field studies in particular struggle to maintain control in a similar way to experimental lab-based studies, and often present this high within-group variability.

Single-case designs offer a useful alternative for the sport and exercise practitioner with practical methods to assess change in a target variable. Sound visual analysis guidelines help practitioners to judge whether the treatment effectively changed the target variable. Visual analysis can be supported using a range of user-friendly statistical techniques. There are also many more advanced techniques available for researchers and practitioners beyond the scope of this book and therefore for further guidance readers are directed to the work of Barlow et al. (2009), Bloom et al. (2009) and Cooper et al. (2007). This book concludes with a summary of the major issues emanating from the book so far along with recommendations for students, researchers and practitioners.

Key points

- Visual analysis is the traditional method for analysing behaviour in single-case research designs.
- Visual analysis has specific rules to guide researchers' and practitioners' decisions about change in a target variable.
- Statistical analysis is proposed as a suitable method to help analyse data from single-case research designs.

Guided study

Your task in this chapter is to locate two studies that have used single-case research designs and explain the type of behavioural assessment used in each study. You'll find examples in the *Journal of Applied Behavior Analysis, The Sport Psychologist, Psychology of Sport and Exercise* and the *Journal of Applied Sport Psychology*. Answer the questions below about each study.

- Was visual analysis and/or statistical analysis used in the study?
- Were decisions rules for visual analysis outlined in each study?
- Using Parsonson and Baer's (1978) heuristic guide to analysis of graphed data, do you think that the authors made an accurate assessment of behaviour change?
- If statistical analysis was used, which statistics were reported? Were they appropriate?
- Did the statistical analysis support or refute the findings from the visual analysis of graphed data?

10

SINGLE-CASE RESEARCH IN SPORT AND EXERCISE

Progress and prospects

In this chapter, we will:

*   re-visit 'small numbers' ('small *n*') research in psychology and explain its history and significance;
*   summarize some key features of single-case research designs and provide a practical checklist to help you evaluate studies in this field;
*   illustrate the main advantages and disadvantages of using single-case research designs in sport and exercise psychology;
*   outline some old challenges for, and new directions in, single-case design research in sport and exercise psychology.

Introduction

In this book, single-case research designs have been discussed primarily from a psychological perspective, which is in keeping with most literature on single-case research designs and our background as sport and exercise psychologists. Therefore, this final chapter focuses on summarizing the main issues surrounding single-case research also from the perspective of sport and exercise psychology. In addition this chapter makes a number of recommendations relevant to other domains in sport and exercise, such as coaching, biomechanics, physiology and nutrition.

The nature and importance of small numbers ('small *n*') research in psychology

Over seventy years ago, Allport (1937) distinguished between two different scientific traditions in psychology – the 'nomothetic' and 'idiographic' approaches.

While the nomothetic approach attempts to establish general laws of behaviour using data obtained from group comparisons, the idiographic approach is concerned mainly with the intensive study of individuals over time. Researchers in the nomothetic tradition advocate the use of controlled laboratory experiments ('group designs') in which different groups of of participants are exposed to different treatment conditions and the performance of the group exposed to the treatment is compared statistically with that of a control (no-treatment) group. By contrast, idiographic investigators tend to use descriptive approaches such as 'case studies' or methods that involve the intensive description and analysis of a single person or instance of a situation (Moran 2011). Although nomothetic and idiographic methodological approaches are best regarded as complementary rather than mutually exclusive, they are often portrayed as being incompatible. For example, Allport (1962) argued that that the uniqueness of people cannot be reduced to, or validly represented by, average values. Similarly, Frank (1986, p. 24) proposed that 'nomothetic science can never escape the individual . . . its findings must eventually be applied to the individual'. Despite these latter objections, the nomothetic tradition has largely held sway in traditional psychological research with its researchers preferring to use group designs rather than case studies. Neverthelesss, as Chapter 2 suggests, there is a venerable tradition of idiographic or 'small *n*' research (i.e., studies involving only one or a handful of participants; Shaughnessy, Zechmeister and Zechmeister 2000) in psychology from the earliest years of the discipline. And because we need to know where we have come *from* in order to find out where we are going *to*, the purpose of this section of the chapter is to trace the history and explain the significance of case-study research in psychology.

As Chapter 1 explains, case-study research has long been used in the natural sciences. For example, in the nineteenth century, Charles Darwin's research on individual bird species (especially Galápagos finches) contributed greatly to the theory of evolution. Similarly, a single-case approach was evident in Donald Johanson's discovery in 1974 of the fossilized remains of the partial skeleton of a female hominid ('Lucy') that had a small brain and had walked upright over three milion years ago. This discovery was immensely significant because it disproved the popular theory that brain enlargement *preceded* the ability to walk upright (Ward 2010). Perhaps not surprisingly, case studies have also played a key role in the development of scientific psychology since the mid- to late nineteenth century. For example, Fechner (1966), who developed a branch of experimental psychology called 'psychophysics' (the scientific study of the relationship between physical stimuli and perceptual experience; Mather 2009), relied on data collected from in-depth studies of a small number of individuals. Using such methods he believed that he had discovered the 'exact science of the functional relations . . . between body and mind' (cited in Schwartz 1987, p. 46). Similarly, as we mentioned in Chapters 1 and 2, Ebbinghaus (1964) conducted perhaps the most famous example of single-case research in psychology when he served as both a participant and an experimenter in his ground-breaking research on verbal learning and memory. Remarkably, he learned about 2,000 lists of nonsense syllables in his research career (Dukes 1965). Another single-case research strategy was used more recently in cognitive psychology by Linton (1975) who extended Ebbinghaus' (1964) research by investigating autobiographical memory processes for daily events over a five-year period using a single participant – herself. Over this period of time, Linton (1975) systematically kept a diary of two events per day. At predetermined intervals, she randomly selected a sample of these items and tried to date them. Two interesting results emerged. First, she displayed an impressive memory for the mundane events in her diary – remembering over 65 per cent of them after three years. Second, the pattern of forgetting that she discovered appeared to be linear, with a slope of about 5 per cent loss of items per year, rather than logarithmic, as Ebbinghaus (1964) had suggested (Baddeley 1997).

Other valuable insights into the mind have come from cognitive psychologists using case studies. For example, Chase and Ericsson (1981) used a single participant ('SF') to study the effects of extensive practice on memory. They trained SF (whose original memory span was about the average of seven units) over 200 practice sessions spanning several months to achieve a remarkable memory span whereby he could recall accurately over *eighty* digits presented randomly! How was this feat accomplished? Interestingly, SF was a keen varsity track athlete who used his knowledge of running times to 'chunk' (or break into smaller, more meaningful units) the digits to be remembered into familiar units. For example, he might break up six digits such as 220416 into two chunks using the time taken to run a marathon (two hours and twenty minutes) followed by that to run a mile (four minutes and sixteen seconds). Remarkably, SF's extraordinary memory skill was confined to numbers only. Thus he was no better than average in his ability to recall long strings of *letters*. The clear implication of this study is that people's memory span can be increased if they practise chunking techniques based on specialist knowledge or personal interest. Overall, SF managed to increase his short-term memory span for digits *tenfold* by practising extensively.

Learning theorists in psychology have also favoured the 'small *n*' research strategy. Indeed, Skinner (1966), in advocating the experimental analysis of behaviour, famously proclaimed that 'instead of studying a thousand rats for one hour each or a hundred rats for 10 hours each, the investigator is more likely to study one rat for a thousand hours' (p. 21). Clearly, Skinner preferred a study with a thousand replications of a *single* participant to one with a thousand participants. Case studies have also been used extensively in cognitive neuropsychology (e.g., Carmazza and McCloskey 1988) to study individual differences in the neurological substrates of cognitive processes. Such case studies can provide vivid, dramatic and compelling insights for the general reader into the minds of patients with bizarre neurological disorders (e.g., see Broks 2004; Campbell 1992; Sacks 1985). For example, Sacks' (1985) best-selling book *The Man Who Mistook His Wife for a Hat* includes the case study of a man with visual agnosia (a condition in which people's ability to recognize objects is impaired) who, literally, seized his wife's head when attempting to put on his hat!

The preceding examples show that idiographic research extends from the earliest days of experimental psychology through learning theory to contemporary studies of perception and cognition. Despite this tradition, Barlow and Nock (2009) pointed out that the nomothetic paradigm has become the dominant method of establishing internal validity (i.e., the extent to which a research method can exclude alternative explanations for the effect of an independent variable) and external validity (i.e., the extent to which the results of a study generalize to other people, groups and settings) in psychological research.

In general, case studies are not only dramatic and evocative but also have at least three advantages as scientific research methods (Shaughnessy et al. 2000). First, they are helpful in describing rare phenomena – for example the neurological impairments identified and compiled by Sacks (1985). Second, case studies of children (e.g., as investigated by Piaget 1952) or of people with emotional problems (e.g., as indicated by Freud 1964) can generate hypotheses about behaviour and experience that can be followed up more systematically in controlled laboratory studies. Finally, case studies can provide data that either challenge prevailing theory (e.g., recall the anthropologist Johanson's 1974 discovery of 'Lucy') or corroborate it (e.g., the theoretical distinction between long-term memory and short-term or working memory was supported by the discovery of a patient, 'H. M', whose immediate memory was intact but who could not put new information into his long-term memory; see Parkin 1999). Unfortunately, despite the preceding strengths, case studies have a number of weaknesses (Shaughnessy et al. 2000). For example, they are vulnerable to biases in data collection and interpretation (e.g., investigators may 'discover' what they expect to find). In addition, because extraneous variables are not controlled in case studies, they do not allow valid inferences to be drawn regarding cause and effect. And that brings us neatly to single-case *experimental* designs – as distinct from case studies. These idiographic methods differ from case studies because, in single-case research, variables are manipulated and repeated measures data are collected and analysed – thereby enabling researchers to draw valid inferences about cause and effect (Ray and Schottelkorb 2010). Clearly, because they are *experimental* rather than correlational in nature, single-case research designs provide greater rigour than that available from other methods such as case studies, correlational investigations or descriptive studies based on surveys. Typically, single-case research designs differ from traditional independent group designs by preferring to look for changes in the target behaviour after the independent variable has been introduced rather than by employing inferential statistics.

Single-case research designs: key features and a reviewer's checklist

As we have explained throughout this book, 'single-case' research designs are a group of (quasi)-experimental methods that grew out of attempts in the applied behaviour analysis tradition (e.g., Leslie and O'Reilly 1999) to understand an individual's behaviour – especially his or her response to an intervention pro-gramme (Kratochwill and Levin 2010). They can be used to study the effect, time course or variability of an independent variable (e.g., an intervention pro-gramme or psychological process) on some designated dependent (outcome) variables. Single-case research is typically used both for theoretical reasons (e.g., to test conceptually derived hypotheses) and for practical reasons (e.g., to validate the efficacy of a specific intervention programme in order to establish evidence-based practice). Overall, according to Horner et al. (2005, p. 165), single-case research is a 'rigorous, scientific methodology used to define basic principles of behaviour and establish evidence-based practices'. In these designs, data are collected on each 'case' and are individually analysed (see Chapter 9). Although single-case designs are also known as '$n = 1$,' single-subject' or 'small n' designs (Ray and Schottelkorb 2010), the term 'single case' does not refer to the *number* of participants in the study – it designates the *procedure* for data collection (Barger-Anderson, Domaracki, Kearney-Vakulick and Kubina 2004). Thus the 'units' in single-case research can be an individual participant, a dyad, a small group or even an institutional population (Kratochwill and Levin 2010).

As is clear from previous chapters, single-case research designs have a number of key features (Horner et al. 2005). First, in these designs the individual participant is the unit of analysis – whether only one participant or multiple participants take part – and each participant serves as his or her own control. Typically, a participant's performance of target variables before the intervention is introduced is compared with performance of these target variables during and/or after the intervention. Second, in order to facilitate rep-lication by future researchers, single-case designs require precise and detailed descriptions of contextual features of the experiment such as the participants and the setting in which data were collected. Third, single-case research requires clear operational definition and continuous measurement of outcome (dependent) variables. Such dependent variables should be selected for their social significance [i.e., their perceived importance to the participant(s)] and should be 'assessed repeatedly within and across phases of the experiment in a time-series fashion' (Kratochwill and Levin 2010, p. 126). Usually, measure-ment of target variables takes place before the start of the intervention under investigation and also during its implementation. Fourth, the independent variable in single-case research must be operationally defined and actively manipulated. Fifth, in order to demonstrate experimental control over a given target behaviour, single-case research requires a baseline comparison condition. In this design, performance of target variables during the baseline (or 'treatment as usual') condition is compared with performance of target variables during and/or after the intervention. Typically, one or more intervention conditions is compared with one or more baseline (non-intervention) conditions and infer-ences are drawn from either a change in the participants between baseline and intervention phases or a differential change between baseline and intervention conditions (Kratochwill and Levin 2010). Such comparisons are usually based on multiple data points. Sixth, in order to demonstrate internal validity (i.e., whether or not an experimental effect has occurred), it is necessary to show that there has been predicted change in the dependent variable as a function of manipulation of the independent variable. Typical strategies to document experimental control include the 'withdrawal' design (A–B–A; described in Chapter 5) and the 'multiple-baseline' design (described in Chapter 6). In the former, a baseline (no-intervention) phase (A) is followed by a treatment phase (B), which is then followed by a return to baseline or reversal phase (A). In the multiple-baseline design, the introduction of the independent variable is staggered at different points in time for each behaviour, participant or setting. If the dependent variable changes only when the treatment is introduced, the effects can be attributed plausibly to that intervention. As we explained previously (see Chapter 6), there are three main types of multiple-baseline designs – those across behaviours, across participants and across settings. It should be noted, however, that multiple-case research designs are based on replication logic – not representative sampling (Smith 1988). However, Kratochwill and Levin (2010) have recently proposed that randomization can be introduced into the various types of single-case designs. Seventh, as Chapter 9 explains, analysis of data in single-case designs is typically based on systematic visual comparison of participants' responses within and across conditions of the study. According to Martin and Pear (2003), this visual inspection pays special attention to variables such as the number of overlapping data points between pre- and post-intervention phases (the fewer the number, the greater the intervention effects), the size of the effects after intervention and the number of times the findings are replicated across participants. Nevertheless, as we explained in Chapter 9, statistical analysis of serially dependent single-case data is possible. For example, time-series analysis allows researchers to evaluate the nature, magnitude and direction of the relationship between variables that are measured at several equidistant points in time (Kinugasa et al. 2004). Interestingly, Callow and Waters (2005) used a statistical procedure called ITSACORR (which analyses single-case data without violating conventional parametric assmptions; see Crosbie 1993) in their investigation of the efficacy of a kinasethetic imagery intervention in enhancing confidence in three professional flat-race jockeys. Results showed that this intervention led to an increase in confidence in two of the three participants in this study. Finally, in common with other experimental designs, single-case research seeks to establish the extent to which its effects generalize adequately to other participants and settings (recall the reference earlier to the term 'external validity').

In Table 10.1 we present a summary of Horner et al.'s (2005) 'quality indicators' of single-case design research in an effort to help you to become a more critical consumer of research in this field.

TABLE 10.1 Evaluating single-case research designs: critical thinking questions

1. Participants	Are participants described in sufficient detail to enable you to replicate the study?
	Is the process by which participants were recruited described sufficiently precisely to enable replication?
2. Dependent variable(s)	Are the dependent variables operationally defined and described with replicable precision?
	Are the dependent variables measured repeatedly over time?
	Is there adequate interobserver agreement on the reliability of dependent variables? (e.g., as measured by correlation coefficients, percentage agreement or Cohen's kappa)
3. Independent variable(s)	Are the indendent variables described sufficiently precisely to facilitate replication?
	What is the evidence in favour of the construct validity of the independent variable?
	Were the independent variables manipulated systematically?
4. Baseline condition	Is the baseline condition described sufficiently precisely to facilitate replication?
	Does the baseline condition describe repeated measurements of a dependent variable?
5. Internal validity	Does the design provide at least three demonstrations of intervention effects at different points in time?
	Do the results of the study present graphs of the performance of individual participants across baseline and treatment phases?
6. External validity	Are the experimental effects replicated across participants and/or settings?
7. Social validity	Is the magnitude of change in the dependent variable resulting from the intervention socially important?

Sources: Based on Horner et al. (2005); Tankersley, Cook and Cook (2008).

Single-case research designs in sport and exercise psychology: some advantages and disadvantages

Although single-case research designs have been used to evaluate clinical interventions and to determine evidence-based practice (Hayes, Barlow and Nelson-Gray 1999) in fields such as clinical psychology, special education (Odom et al. 2003), school psychology (e.g., Skinner 2004), play therapy (Ray and Schottelkorb 2010) and rehabilitation psychology (e.g., Callahan and Barisa 2005), they have not been widely employed in sport and exercise psychology. To illustrate, Martin et al. (2004) reported that during the three decades between 1974 and 2004, single-case research designs averaged only 0.6, 1.2 and 2.2 published papers per year respectively. The infrequency of usage of single-case research in sport and exercise psychology is probably attributable to the fact that, historically, group design methodology has been the 'gold standard' for investigating causal relationships between independent and dependent variables (Kratochwill and Levin 2010; Smith 1988).

Despite their relative neglect, single-case designs have at least six features that indicate their suitability for use in sport and exercise psychology research. First, they allow researchers to intensively evaluate changes in individual participants' target variables (e.g., behaviour) over time that may be masked by the average scores calculated in randomized group designs. This sensitivity to temporal dynamics is important because, in elite sport, subtle changes in speed of performance from baseline to the post-intervention phase may be practically rather than statistically significant. For example, the difference between the 100-m sprint time of 2008 Olympic gold medallist Usain Bolt (Jamaica; 9.69 seconds) and fourth-placed Churandy Martina (Netherlands Antilles; 9.93 seconds) was only 0.24 seconds – a small time difference but one that was highly important in this race. More generally, as you may recall, this issue of the difference between statistical significance and meaningful significance in single-case research was addressed in Chapter 3. Briefly, it refers to the fact that, although an intervention may not produce a statistically significant difference in an athlete's performance, it may be perceived as being *practically* important to the athlete concerned.

Second, single-case research designs are especially useful for the task of empirically validating mental skills interventions for athletes. For example, Thelwell, Greenlees and Weston (2006) used a multiple-baseline across-participants design to assess the effectiveness of a psychological skills intervention that had been developed to improve three specific components of a soccer midfield player's performance – accuracy of 'first touch' of the ball, pass completion percentage and tackle success percentage. Using an intervention that included training in relaxation, mental imagery and self-talk, and having assessed targeted performance across nine competitive matches, these authors found small experimental effects for four of the five football players in the sample. Third, as explained in earlier chapters, because single-case research designs do not use independent control groups, they are useful for circumventing any ethical issues that may arise if an intervention that is known to be effective (e.g., one based on mental practice; see Driskell, Copper and Moran 1994; Moran 2011) is either withheld altogether or withdrawn after it has been introduced initially. A fourth aspect of single-case research designs that makes them suitable for use in sport and exercise settings is that they facilitate analysis of differences *among* 'non-responders' (i.e., participants whose target variables remain unaffected or are made worse by the intervention under investigation) as well as *between* 'non-responders' and 'responders' (i.e., participants who benefit from the intervention being administered; Horner et al. 2005). In other words, single-case designs enable researchers to detect successful effects for individuals whose changes in variables (i.e., behaviour) may have been masked in a group design. For example, from their analysis of the results of their single-case study, Thelwell et al. (2006) suggested a possible reason why one of their participants did not show improvements in all of the dependent variables that they measured. Specifically, not all midfield players play exactly the same roles in their teams. Thus, although the requirement of 'good tackling ability' may apply to a defensive midfield player, it does not apply as strongly to attacking midfield players. So the authors concluded that 'from an applied perspective, practitioners need to be aware of the role-specific requirements of the performers with whom they work' (p. 267). More generally, as Martin et al. (2004) noted, the fact that sport psychology journals tend to publish single-case research studies that report *few* or *no* experimental effects may be helpful for practitioners in the field because it provides published data on weak interventions. Fifth, multiple-baseline single-case designs allow investigators to 'individualize' interventions (Cumming and Ramsey 2009) or to tailor aspects of the intervention to the unique requirements of individual participants. To illustrate, Callow and Waters (2005) examined the efficacy of a six-session kinaesthetic (or 'feeling-oriented') imagery intervention (administered twice a week for three weeks) in increasing the confidence of three professional flat-race jockeys. During this intervention, each participant received five individualized imagery 'scripts' (or sets of instructions) to take account of the particular horse that they were riding and/or the location of the race that they were being asked to imagine. Using a multiple-baseline across-participants design, the authors discovered that, as expected, the imagery intervention increased confidence among the jockeys – but only for two of the three participants in the study. More generally, as Kinugasa et al. (2004) pointed out, single-case research designs appeal to applied researchers and practitioners because they are 'sufficiently flexible to accommodate the changing needs of the individual studied' (p. 1037). Finally, because single-case research can be conducted with minimal changes to athletes' normal training and competitive programmes, their ecological validity is high (Jones 1996).

Despite the preceding advantages, single-case research designs have a number of limitations that need to be acknowledged (Jones 1996; Shaughnessy et al. 2000). First, most single-case research designs are insensitive to interaction effects. In other words, they cannot evaluate the possibility that the effect of a given independent variable on a specific outcome may depend on its interaction with another independent variable. Second, because statistical tests are not normally conducted on data yielded by single-case research designs, it is difficult to provide any quantitative index of confidence in the generalizability of the results. More generally, the issue of data analysis in single-case research has been controversial. For example, as Callahan and Barisa (2005, p. 25) noted, 'it is difficult to obtain guidance on how many observations are sufficient for a reasonable sampling, what constitutes a trend, or how much change is needed to conclude that some effect has in fact occurred'. Third, it can be difficult to interpret the effects of a treatment intervention if the baseline data show excessive variability. For this reason, researchers need to establish stable baseline measurements of all dependent variables before the intervention is introduced. Finally, although single-case studies are helpful in exploring experimental effects at an *individual* level, their capacity to generalize findings validly to other participants and settings is questionable. Nevertheless, several essential criteria required to produce rigorous studies (e.g., adequate internal and external validity, experimental control, and replication) are evident in single-case research designs.

Single-case research designs: old challenges and new directions

Throughout this book we have emphasized the potential utility of single-case designs for researchers and practitioners in sport and exercise settings. In particular, these designs not only are helpful in identifying small but significant changes in individual athletes' and exercisers' performances over time but also can be used to evaluate interventions and hence to establish cost-effective, evidence-based practice – a requirement that is increasingly emphasized in the domain of applied sport and exercise psychology (e.g., see Hemmings and Holder 2009). In passing, it is notable that the scientist-practitioner model for clinical psychologists postulated at the Boulder Conference in 1949 (see Barlow et al. 1984) advocated that professionals in this field should be not only consumers of new research findings and evaluators of interventions through empirical methods but also investigators who produce data from their own 'laboratory' to inform colleagues. Clearly, such requirements are equally applicable to sport and exercise scientists.

What old challenges and new directions may be identified in single-case research in sport and exercise psychology? First, based on the review by Martin et al. (2004), it is clear that single-case researchers in this field have not used enough elite athletes in their studies. For example, only two of the 222 participants who took part in forty selected studies reviewed by Martin et al. (2004) were international-level sports performers – and *none* was a professional athlete. This relative neglect of elite athletes by researchers is not confined to single-case research. Indeed, there has been a dearth of studies in the discipline that evaluate mental practice interventions on elite athletes in field settings (Moran 2011). Clearly a key new direction for future single-case researchers is to incorporate more elite athletes into their studies (e.g., Barker and Jones 2008). A second persistent challenge in single-case research is to identify the most effective components of mental skills interventions. In the past, as noted by Moran (2011), applied sport psychology consultants have tended to use broadly similar 'packages' of psychological strategies (e.g., goal-setting, self-talk) to address a variety of different athletic problems. This 'one size fits all' approach to implementing psychological skills interventions with athletes is regrettable because it fails to shed light on underlying psychological processes. As Martin et al. (2004) concluded when referring to mental skills intervention packages using goal-setting, self-talk and imagery, 'it is not clear that all components contributed to the effectiveness of the package' (p. 277). Fortunately, the challenge of identifying effective components of interventions has been accepted by researchers such as Thelwell et al. (2006) who have conducted rigorous componential analyses of the processes in question. Additional componential analyses need to be conducted to evaluate the efficacy of psychological interventions in sport and exercise research. A third challenge facing single-case researchers in sport and exercise psychology is methodological – how to incorporate statistical developments (e.g., Callahan and Barisa 2005) and sampling innovations (e.g., Kratochwill and Levin 2010) in other areas into traditional designs in this field. This incorporation is necessary because the qualitative nature of traditional single-case analysis is sometimes regarded with suspicion by researchers trained in quantitative analysis of group designs.

Summary

We began this chapter by distinguishing between the nomothetic and idiographic methodological approaches in psychology and by explaining the nature and significance of 'small numbers' ('small n') idiographic research in psychology. We also traced the history of case-study research in this discipline. In the next section, we highlighted some key features of single-case research designs and presented a checklist of questions to help in evaluating research using this method. We then reviewed the main advantages and disadvantages of single-case research designs in sport and exercise psychology. Finally, we discussed some old challenges for, and potentially fruitful new directions in, single-case design research in this discipline.

Overall, this book is the first of its kind to bring single-case research methods to the domain of sport and exercise. The major focus of the book has been exploring single-case research methods from the perspective of sport and exercise psychology, primarily because of our expertise in this area. However, despite this psychological 'feel' our ultimate aim in compiling and publishing this book was to endorse the application of single-case procedures by sport and exercise science researchers and practitioners (including coaches, biomechanists, physiologists, nutritionists). Our endorsement of single-case methods was done for a number of reasons. First, these methods have largely been underused in sport and exercise (aside from sport and exercise psychology) in comparison with other applied domains (e.g., psychology, social work, education). Second, the methods are theoretically neutral and thus can easily be imported into applied settings. Third, such methods can assist sport and exercise researchers and practitioners in developing the literature on evidence-based practice. Finally, the methods provide a framework for determining intervention effectiveness in the current climate of accountability. In sum, we now recommend the development of innovative research training and research projects using single-case methods. Both of these developments should encourage the adoption and use of single-case methods by those involved in sport and exercise.

Key points

- External validity is when the results of a particular study can be applied to participants, behaviours or settings beyond a specific study. If a study is high in external validity data are generalizable to large populations.
- Data are said to be statistically significant when the outcome would occur less than 5 per cent of the time if the populations were identical.
- Meaningful significance is when a noticeable real-world change in a participant's target variables is observed (e.g., sport performance).
- 'Idiographic' describes the study of the individual, who is seen as an entity, with properties setting him/her apart from other individuals.
- Nomothetic is more the study of a cohort of individuals. Here the participant is seen as representing a class or population and their corresponding personality traits and behaviours.

Guided study

Based upon your reading of Chapter 10 please take some time to respond to the following review questions:

- Explain the history of case-study research and its importance for practitioners and researchers in sport and exercise.
- Outline the key features of single-case research designs.
- Outline the advantages and disadvantages of single-case research designs.
- Outline future directions for the use of single-case research methods in sport and exercise.

REFERENCES

Abelson, R. P. (1985). A variance explanation paradox: When a little is a lot. *Psychological Bulletin, 97*, 128–132.

Agras, W. S., Leitenberg, H., Barlow, D. H. and Thomson, L. E. (1969). Instructions and reinforcement in the modification of neurotic behavior. *American Journal of Psychiatry, 125*, 1435–1439.

Alberto, P. A. and Troutman, A. C. (1999). *Applied behavior analysis for teachers* (5th edn). Columbus, OH: Merrill.

Allen, K. D. (1998). The use of an enhanced simplified habit-reversal procedure to reduce disruptive outburst during athletic performance. *Journal of Applied Behavior Analysis, 31*, 489–492.

Allen, K. D. and Evans, J. H. (2001). Exposure-based treatment to control excessive blood glucose monitoring. *Journal of Applied Behavior Analysis, 34*, 497–500.

Allison, M. G. and Ayllon, T. (1980). Behavioral coaching in the development of skills in football, gymnastics, and tennis. *Journal of Applied Behavior Analysis, 13*, 297–314.

Allport, G. W. (1937). *Personality: A psychological interpretation*. New York: Holt.

Allport, G. W. (1962). The general and the unqiue in psychological science. *Journal of Personality, 30*, 405–422.

Andersen, M. B., McCullagh, P. and Wilson, G. J. (2007). But what do the numbers really tell us?: Arbitrary metrics and effect size reporting in sport psychology research. *Journal of Sport & Exercise Psychology, 29*, 664–672.

Anderson, G. and Kirkpatrick, M. A. (2002). Variable effects of a behavioral treatment package on the performance of inline roller speed skaters. *Journal of Applied Behavior Analysis, 35*, 195–198.

Anderson, A. G., Miles, A., Mahoney, C. and Robinson, P. (2002). Evaluating the effectiveness of applied sport psychology practice: Making the case for a case study approach. *The Sport Psychologist, 16*, 432–453.

Arco, L. (2008). Neurobehavioral treatment for obsessive-compulsive disorder in an adult with traumatic brain injury. *Neuropsychological Rehabilitation, 18*, 109–124.

Aronson, E., Ellsworth, P. C., Carlsmith, J. M. and Gonzales, M. H. (1990). *Methods of research in social psychology* (2nd edn). New York: McGraw-Hill.

Baddeley, A. (1997). *Human memory: Theory and practice* (revised edition). Hove, East Sussex: Psychology Press.

Baer, D. M., Wolf, M. M. and Risley, T. R. (1968). Some current dimensions of applied behavior analysis. *Journal of Applied Behavior Analysis, 1*, 91–97.

Bailey, D. B. (1984). Effects of lines of progress and semilogarithmic charts on ratings of charted data. *Journal of Applied Behavior Analysis, 17*, 359–365.

Bailey, J. S. and Birch, M. R. (2002). *Research methods in applied behaviour analysis*. London: Sage.

Bar-Eli, M., Dreshman, R., Blumenstein, B. and Weinstein, Y. (2002). The effect of mental training with biofeedback on the performance of young swimmers. *Applied Psychology: An International Review, 51*, 567–581.

Barger-Anderson, P., Domaracki, J. W., Kearney-Vakulick and Kubina, R. M., Jr. (2004). Multiple baseline designs: The use of single-case experimental design in literacy. *Reading Improvement, 41*, 217–225.

Barker, J. B. and Jones, M. V. (2006). Using hypnosis, technique refinement, and self-modelling to enhance self-efficacy: A case study in cricket. *The Sport Psychologist, 20*, 94–110.

Barker, J. B. and Jones, M. V. (2008). The effects of hypnosis on self-efficacy, positive and negative affect and sport performance: A case study from professional English soccer. *Journal of Clinical Sport Psychology, 2*, 127–147.

Barker, J. B., Jones, M. V. and Greenlees, I. (2010). Assessing the immediate and maintained effects of hypnosis on self-efficacy and soccer wall-volley performance. *Journal of Sport & Exercise Psychology, 32*, 243–252.

Barlow, D. H. and Hayes, S. C. (1979). Alternating treatments design: One strategy for comparing the effects of two treatments in a single subject. *Journal of Applied Behavior Analysis, 12*, 199–210.

Barlow, D. H. and Hersen, M. (1984). *Single-case experimental designs: Strategies for studying behavior change* (2nd edn). New York: Pergamon Press.

Barlow, D. H. and Nock, M. K. (2009). Why can't we be more idiographic in our research? *Perspectives on Psychological Science, 4*, 19–21.

Barlow, D. H., Hayes, S. C. and Nelson, R. M. (1984). *The scientist practitioner: Research and accountability in clinical educational settings*. New York: Pergamon.

Barlow, D. H., Nock, M. K. and Hersen, M. (2009). *Single-case experimental designs: Strategies for studying behavior change* (3rd edn). New York: Pearson

Baron, R. A. and Richardson, D. R. (1994). *Human aggression*. New York: Plenum Press.

Barrett, T. (2005). Effects of co-operative learning on the performance of sixth-grade physical education students. *Journal of Teaching in Physical Education, 24*, 88–102.

Bates, P., Renzaglia, A. and Clees, T. J. (1980). Improving the work performance of severely/profoundly retarded young adults: The use of a changing criterion procedural design. *Education and Training of the Mentally Retarded, 15*, 95–104.

Beck, A. T., Steer, R. A. and Brown, G. K. (1996). *Manual for the Beck depression inventory (BDI-II)* (2nd edn). San Antonio, TX: Psychological Association.

Bengali, M. K. and Ottenbacher, K. J. (1998). The effect of autocorrelation on the results of visually analysing data from single-subject designs. *American Journal of Occupational Therapy, 52*, 650–655.

Birnbrauer, J. S. (1981). External validity and experimental investigation of individual behavior. *Analysis and Intervention in Developmental Disabilities, 1*, 117–132.

Blampied, N. M. (2000). Single-case research designs: A neglected alternative. *American Psychologist, 55*, 960.

Blanton, H. and Jaccard, J. (2006). Arbitrary metrics in psychology. *American Psychologist, 61*, 27–41.

Bloom, M., Fischer, J. and Orme, J. G. (2009). *Evaluating practice: Guidelines for the accountable professional* (6th edn). New York: Allyn & Bacon.

Boring, E. G. (1954). The nature and the history of experimental control. *American Journal of Psychology, 67*, 573–589.

Boutcher, S. H. (1990). The role of performance routines in sport. In J. G. Jones and L. Hardy (eds) *Stress and performance in sport* (pp. 231–245). Chichester: John Wiley.

Boyer, E., Miltenberger, R. G., Batsche, C. and Fogel, V. (2009). Video modelling by experts with video feedback to enhance gymnastics skills. *Journal of Applied Behavior Analysis, 42*, 855–860.

Broks, P. (2004). *Into the silent land: Travels in neuropsychology*. New York: Grove Press.

Brossart, D. F., Meythaler, J. M., Parker, R. I., McNamara, J. and Elliott, T. R. (2008). Advanced regression methods for single-case designs: Studying propranolol in the treatment for agitation associated with traumatic brain injury. *Rehabilitation Psychology, 53*, 357–369.

Browning, R. A. (1967). A same-subject design for simultaneous comparison of three reinforcement contingencies. *Behavior Therapy, 5*, 237–243.

Browning, R. M. and Stover, D. D. (1971). *Behavior modification in child treatment*. Chicago: Aldine.

Brustad, R. J. (2002). Qualitative research approaches. In T. S. Horn (ed.) *Advances in sport psychology* (pp. 31–43). Champaign, IL; Human Kinetics.

Bryan, A. J. (1987). Single-subject designs for evaluation of sport psychology interventions. *The Sport Psychologist, 1*, 283–292.

Burton, D. (1989). Winning isn't everything: Examining the impact of performance goals on collegiate swimmers' cognitions and performance. *The Sport Psychologist, 3*, 105–132.

Butler, R. J. (1989). Psychological preparation of Olympic boxers. In J. Kremer and W. Crawford (eds) *The psychology of sport: Theory and practice* (pp. 74–84). Belfast: BPS Northern Ireland Branch, occasional paper.

Butler, R. J. and Hardy, L. (1992). The performance profile: Theory and application. *The Sport Psychologist, 6*, 253–264.

Callahan, C. D. and Barisa, M. T. (2005). Statistical process control and rehabilitation outcome: The single-subject design reconsidered. *Rehabilitation Psychology, 50*, 24–33.

Callow, N. and Waters, A. (2005). The effect of kinaesthetic imagery on the sport confidence of flat-race horse jockeys. *Psychology of Sport and Exercise, 6*, 443–459.

Callow, N., Hardy, L. and Hall, C. (2001). The effects of a motivational general-mastery imagery intervention on the sport confidence of high-level badminton players. *Research Quarterly for Exercise and Sport, 72*, 389–400.

Calmels, C., Berthoumieux, C. and d'Arripe-Longueville, F. (2004). Effects of an imagery training program on selective attention of national softball players. *The Sport Psychologist, 18*, 272–296.

Cameron, M. J., Shapiro, R. and Ainsleigh, S. A. (2005). Bicycle riding: Pedaling made possible through positive behavioral interventions. *Journal of Positive Behavior Interventions, 7*, 153–158.

Campbell, D. T. and Stanley, J. C. (1963). *Experimental and quasi-experimental designs for research*. Boston: Houghton-Mifflin.

Campbell, R. (ed.) (1992). *Mental lives: Case studies in cognition*. Oxford: Blackwell.

Carmazza, A. and McCloskey, M. (1988). The case for single-patient studies. *Cognitive Neuropsychology, 5*, 517–528.

Carr, J. E. (2005). Recommendations for reporting multiple-baseline designs across-participants. *Behavioral Interventions, 20*, 219–224.

Chaddock, R. E. (1925). *Principles and methods of statistics*. Boston: Houghton-Mifflin.

Chase, W. G. and Ericsson, K. A. (1981). Skilled memory. In J. R. Anderson (ed.), *Cognitive skills and their acquisition* (pp. 141–189). Hillsdale, NJ: Erlbaum.

Clark-Carter, D. (2009). *Quantitative psychological research: The complete student's companion*. Hove: Psychology Press.

Cohen, J. (1988). *Statistical power analysis for the behavioral sciences* (2nd edn). Hillsdale, NJ: Erlbaum.

Collins, D., Morriss, C. and Trower, J. (1999). Getting it back: A case study of skill recovery in an elite athlete. *The Sport Psychologist, 13*, 288–298.

Conroy, D. E., Kaye, M. P. and Schantz, L. H. (2002). Quantitative research methodology. In T. S. Horn (ed.) *Advances in sport psychology* (pp. 15–30). Champaign, IL; Human Kinetics.

Cooper, J. O., Heron, T. E. and Heward, W. L. (2007). *Applied behavior analysis* (2nd edn). Upper Saddle River, NJ: Pearson/Merrill Prentice Hall.

Critchfield, T. S. and Vargas, E. A. (1991). Self-recording, instructions, and public graphing: Effects on swimming in the absence of coach verbal interaction. *Behavior Modification, 15*, 95–112.

Crosbie, J. (1993). Interrupted time-series analysis with brief single-subject data. *Journal of Consulting and Clinical Psychology, 61*, 966–974.

Crosbie, J. (1995). Interrupted time-series analysis with short series: Why it is problematic: How it can be improved. In J. M. Gottman and G. Sackett (eds) *The analysis of change* (pp. 361–395). Hillsdale, NJ: Erlbaum.

Crouch, D., Ward, P. and Patrick, C. (1997). The effects of peer-mediated accountability on task accomplishment during volley-ball drills in elementary physical education. *Journal of Teaching in Physical Education, 17*, 26–39.

Crowne, D. P. and Marlowe, D. (1960). A new scale of social desirability independent of psychopathology. *Journal of Consulting Psychology, 24*, 349–354.

Cumming, J. and Ramsey, R. (2009). Imagery interventions in sport. In S. D. Mellalieu and S. Hanton (eds) *Advances in applied sport psychology: A review* (pp. 5–36). London: Routledge.

Davis, P. A. and Sime, W. E. (2005). Toward a psychophysiology of performance: Sport psychology principles dealing with anxiety. *International Journal of Stress Management, 12*, 363–378.

Deese, J. (1972). *Psychology as science and art*. New York: Harcourt Brace Jovanovich.

DeLuca, R. V. and Holborn, S. W. (1992). Effects of a variable-ratio reinforcement schedule with changing criteria on exercise in obese and nonobese boys. *Journal of Applied Behavior Analysis, 25*, 671–679.

DeProspero, A. and Cohen, S. (1979). Inconsistent visual analysis of intra-subject data. *Journal of Applied Behavior Analysis, 12*, 573–579.

Driskell, J. E., Copper, C. and Moran, A. (1994). Does mental practice enhance performance? *Journal of Applied Psychology, 79*, 481–492.

Duda, J. L. (ed.). (1998). *Advances in sport and exercise psychology measurement*. Morgantown, WV: Fitness Information Technology.

Dukes, W. F. (1965). N = 1. *Psychological Bulletin, 64*, 74–79.

Ebbinghaus, H. (1964). *Memory: A contribution to experimental psychology*. New York: Dover. First published in 1885.

Edgington, E. S. (1966). Statistical inference and nonrandom samples. *Psychological Bulletin, 66*, 485–487.

Edgington, E. S. (1972). N = 1 experiments: Hypothesis testing. *The Canadian Psychologist, 2,* 121–134.

Edinger, J. D. (1978). Modification of smoking behavior in a correctional institution. *Journal of Clinical Psychology, 34,* 991–998.

Fechner, G. (1966). *Elements of psychophysics* (Vol. 1). New York: Holt, Rinehart & Winston. First published in 1860.

Ferron, J. (2002). Reconsidering the use of the general linear model with single-case data. *Behavior Research Methods, Instruments, and Computers, 34,* 324–331.

Fisher, R. A. (1925). *Statistical methods for research workers.* Edinburgh: Oliver & Boyd.

Fisher, R. A. (1935). *The design of experiments.* Edinburgh: Oliver & Boyd.

Flood, W. A. and Wilder, D. A. (2004). The use of differential reinforcement and fading to increase time away from a caregiver in a child with separation anxiety disorder. *Education and Treatment of Children, 27,* 1–8.

Foxx, R. M. and Rubinoff, A. (1979). Behavioral treatment of caffeinism: Reducing excessive coffee drinking. *Journal of Applied Behavior Analysis, 12,* 335–344.

Frank, I. (1986). Psychology as a science: Resolving the idiographic-nomothetic controversy. In J. Valsiner (ed.) *The individual subject and scientific psychology* (pp. 17–36). New York: Plenum Press.

Franklin, R. D., Allison, D. B. and Gorman, B. S. (1996). *Design and analysis of single-case research.* London: Psychology Press.

Franklin, R. D., Gorman, B. S., Beasley, T. M. and Allison, D. B. (1996). Graphical display and visual analysis. In R. D. Franklin, D. B. Allison and B. S. Gorman (eds) *Design and analysis of single-case research* (pp. 119–158). London: Psychology Press.

Freeman, P., Rees, T. and Hardy, L. (2009). An intervention to increase social support and improve performance. *Journal of Applied Sport Psychology, 21,* 186–200.

Freud, S. (1964). *New introductory lectures on psychoanalysis* (ed. and trans. J. Strachey). New York: Norton. First published in 1933.

Friman, P. C. (2009). Behavior assessment. In D. Barlow, M. Nock and M. Hersen (eds), *Single case experimental designs: Strategies for studying behavior change* (3rd edn) (pp. 99–134). Boston, MA: Allyn & Bacon.

Furlong, M. J. and Wampold, B. (1981). Visual analysis of single-subject studies by school psychologists. *Psychology in the Schools, 18,* 80–86.

Furlong, M. J. and Wampold, B. (1982). Intervention effects and relative variation as dimensions in experts' use of visual inference. *Journal of Applied Behavior Analysis, 15,* 415–421.

Gale, E. A. M. (2004). The Hawthorne studies – a fable for our times? *Quarterly Journal of Medicine, 97,* 439–449.

Galvan, Z. J. and Ward, P. (1998). Effects of public posting on inappropriate on-court behaviors by collegiate tennis players. *The Sport Psychologist, 12,* 419–426.

Ganz, J. B. and Flores, M. M. (2008). Effects of the use of visual strategies in play groups for children with autism spectrum disorders and their peers. *Journal of Autism and Developmental Disorders, 39,* 75–83.

Ganz, J. B. and Flores, M. M. (2009). The effectiveness of direct instruction for teaching language to children with autism spectrum disorders: Identifying materials. *Journal of Autism and Developmental Disorders, 39,* 75–83

Gardner, F. and Moore, Z. (2006). *Clinical sport psychology.* Champaign, IL: Human Kinetics.

Gergen, K. J. (1991). *The saturated self: Dilemmas of identity in contemporary life.* New York: Basic Books.

Gliner, J. A., Morgan, G. A. and Leech, N. L. (2009). *Research methods in applied settings: An integrated approach to design and analysis* (2nd edn). London: Routledge.

Goetz, E. M., Holmberg, M. C. and LeBlanc, J. M. (1975). Differential reinforcement of other behavior and noncontingent reinforcement as control procedures during the modification of a preschooler's compliance. *Journal of Applied Behavior Analysis*, 8, 77–82.

Goode, W. J. and Hatt, P. K. (1952). The case study. In W. J. Goode and P. K. Hatt (eds) *Methods of social research* (pp. 330–340). New York: McGraw-Hill.

Gorski, J. A. B. and Westbrook, A. C. (2004). Use of differential reinforcement to treat medical non-compliance in a pediatric patient with leukocyte adhesion deficiency. *Pediatric Rehabilitation, 5*, 29–35.

Gottman, J. M. (1981). *Time-series analysis: A comprehensive introduction for social scientist*. Cambridge: Cambridge University Press.

Gottman, J. M. and Rushe, R. H. (1994). The analysis of change: Issues, fallacies, and new ideas. *Journal of Consulting and Clinical Psychology, 61*, 907–910.

Gould, D. (1993). Goal-setting for peak performance. In J. M. Williams (ed.), *Applied sport psychology: Personal growth to peak performance* (pp. 158–169). Mountain View, CA: Mayfield.

Gregory, R. L. (2004). Falsification. In R. L. Gregory (ed.) *The Oxford companion to the mind* (pp. 337–338). New York: Oxford University Press.

Griffith, C. R. (1926). *The psychology of coaching: A study of coaching methods from the point of psychology*. New York: Scribner's.

Griffith, C. R. (1928). *Psychology of athletics: A general survey for athletes and coaches*. New York: Scribner's.

Grindstaff, J. S. and Fisher, L. A. (2006). Sport psychology consultants' experience of using hypnosis in their practice: An exploratory investigation. *The Sport Psychologist, 20*, 368–386.

Haddad, K. and Tremayne, P. (2009). The effects of centering on the free-throw shooting performance of young athletes. *The Sport Psychologist, 23*, 118–136.

Hall, R. V. and Fox, R. G. (1977). Changing-criterion designs: An alternate applied behavior analysis procedure. In B. C. Etzel, J. M. LeBlanc and D. M. Baer (eds) *New developments in behavioral research: Theory, method, and application* (pp. 151–166). Hillsdale, NJ: Erlbaum.

Hanton, S. and Jones, G. (1999). The effects of a multimodal intervention program on performers: II. Training the butterflies to fly in formation. *The Sport Psychologist, 13*, 22–41.

Harbst, K. B., Ottenbacher, K. J. and Harris, S. R. (1991). Interrater reliability of therapists' judgements of graphed data. *Physical Therapy, 71*, 107–115.

Hartmann, D. P. and Hall, R. V. (1976). The changing-criterion design. *Journal of Applied Behavior Analysis, 9*, 527–532.

Harvey, M. T., May, M. E. and Kennedy, C. H. (2004). Nonconcurrent multiple-baseline designs and the evaluation of educational systems. *Journal of Behavioral Education, 13*, 267–276.

Harwood, C. G. and Swain, A. B. (2002). The development and activation of achievement goals in tennis: II. A player, parent and coach intervention. *The Sport Psychologist, 16*, 111–138.

Haskell, W. L., Lee, I.-M., Pate, R. R., Powell, K. E., Blair, S. N., Franklin, B. A., Macera, C. A., Heath, G. W., Thompson, P. D. and Bauman, A. (2007). Physical activity and public health: Updated recommendation for adults from the American College of

Sports Medicine and the American Heart Association. *Medicine and Science in Sport and Exercise, 39*, 1423–1434,

Hawkins, R. P. (1979). The functions of assessment: Implications for selection and development of devices for assessing repertoires in clinical, educational, and other settings. *Journal of Applied Behavior Analysis, 12*, 501–516.

Hawkins, R. P. and Dobes, R. W. (1977). Behavioral definitions in applied behavior analysis: Explicit or implicit? In B. C. Etzel, J. M. LeBlanc and D. M. Baer (eds), *New developments in behavioral research: Theory, method, and application* (pp. 167–188). Hillsdale, NJ: Erlbaum.

Hayes, S. C. (1981). Single-case research designs and empirical clinical practice. *Journal of Consulting and Clinical Psychology, 49*, 193–211.

Hayes, S. C., Barlow, D. H. and Nelson-Gray, R. O. (1999). *The scientist practitioner: Research and accountability in the age of managed care* (2nd edn). Boston, MA: Allyn & Bacon.

Hazen, A., Johnstone, C., Martin, G. L. and Srikameswaren, S. (1990). A videotaping feedback package for improving skills of youth competitive swimmers. *The Sport Psychologist, 4*, 213–227

Hemmings, B. and Holder, T. (2009). *Applied sport psychology: A case-based approach.* Oxford: Wiley-Blackwell.

Hersen, M. and Barlow, D. H. (1976). *Single-case experimental designs: Strategies for studying behaviour change.* New York: Pergamon.

Heyman, S. R. (1987). Research interventions in sport psychology: Issues encountered in working with an amateur boxer. *The Sport Psychologist, 1*, 208–223.

Hogg, M. A. and Vaughan, G. M. (2008). *Social psychology* (5th edn). Harlow: Prentice Hall.

Holcombe, A., Wolery, M. and Gast, D. L. (1994). Comparative single-subject research: Description of designs and discussion of problems. *Topics in Early Childhood Special Education, 14*, 119–145.

Horner, R. D. and Baer, D. M. (1978). Multiple-probe technique: A variation of the multiple-baseline. *Journal of Applied Behavior Analysis, 11*, 189–196.

Horner, R. M., Carr, E. G., Halle, J., McGee, G., Odom, S. and Wolery, M. (2005). The use of single-subject reesarch to identify evidence-based practice in special education. *Exceptional Children, 71*, 165–179.

Houle, T. T. (2009). Statistical analyses for single-case experimental designs. In D. Barlow, M. Nock and M. Hersen (eds), *Single case experimental designs: Strategies for studying behavior change* (3rd edn) (pp. 271–305). Boston, MA: Allyn & Bacon.

Hrycaiko, D. W. and Martin, G. L. (1996). Applied research studies with single-subject designs: Why so few? *Journal of Applied Sport Psychology, 8*, 183–199.

Huitema, B. E. (2004). Analysis of interrupted time-series experiments using ITSE: A critique. *Understanding Statistics, 3*, 27–46.

Huitema, B. E. and McKean, J. W. (2000). Design specification issues in time-series intervention models. *Educational and Psychological Measurement, 60*, 38–58.

Hume, K. M., Martin, G. L., Gonzalez, P., Cracklen, C. and Genthon, S. (1985). A self-monitoring feedback package for improving freestyle figure skating practice. *Journal of Sport Psychology, 7*, 335–345.

Ittenbach, R. F. and Lawhead, W. F. (1996). Historical and philosophical foundations of single-case research. In R. D. Franklin, D. B. Allison and B. S. Gorman (eds) *Design and analysis of single-case research* (pp. 13–39). New York: Psychology Press.

Jaccard, J. and Becker, M. A. (1990). *Statistics for the behavioral sciences* (2nd edn). Belmont, CA: Wadsworth Publishing.

Johnston, J. M. and Pennypacker, H. S. (1993). *Strategies and tactics of behavioral research* (2nd edn). Hillsdale, NJ: Erlbaum.

Johnston, J. M. and Pennypacker, H. S. (2009). *Strategies and tactics of behavioral research* (3rd edn). New York: Routledge.

Jones, G. (1993). The role of performance profiling in cognitive behavioral interventions in sport. *The Sport Psychologist, 7*, 160–172.

Jones, G. and Swain, A. B. J. (1992). Intensity and direction dimensions of competitive state anxiety and relationships with competitiveness. *Perceptual and Motor Skills, 74*, 467–472.

Jones, M. V. (2003). Controlling emotions in sport. *The Sport Psychologist, 17*, 471–486.

Jones, T. (1996). The advantages/disadvantages of using idiographic multiple baseline designs with elite athletes. In C. Robson, B. Cripps and H. Steinberg (eds) *Quality and quantity: Research methods in sport and exercise psychology* (pp. 10–13). Leciester: British Psychological Society.

Jordan, J., Singh, N. N. and Repp, A. (1989). An evaluation of gentle teaching and visual screening in the reduction of stereotypy. *Journal of Applied Behavior Analysis, 22*, 9–22.

Kadushin, A. (1972). *The social work interview.* London: Columbia University Press.

Kahneman, D. and Tversky, A. (1973). On the psychology of prediction. *Psychological Review, 80*, 237–251.

Kahng, S. W., Boscoe, J. H. and Byrne, S. (2003). The use of an escape contingency and a token economy to increase food acceptance. *Journal of Applied Behavior Analysis, 36*, 349–353.

Katz, J. and Hemmings, B. (2009). *Counselling skills handbook for the sport psychologist.* Leicester: British Psychological Society.

Kazdin, A. E. (1977). Assessing the clinical or applied significance of behavior change through social validation. *Behavior Modification, 1*, 427–452.

Kazdin, A. E. (1978). *History of behavior modification: Experimental foundations of contemporary research.* Baltimore: University Park Press.

Kazdin, A. E. (1982). *Single-case research designs: Method for clinical and applied settings.* New York: Oxford University Press.

Kazdin, A. E. (1994). *Behavior modification in applied settings* (5th edn). Pacific Grove, CA: Brooks/Cole.

Kazdin, A. E. (ed.) (2003). *Methodological issues and strategies in clinical research* (3rd edn). Washington, DC: American Psychological Association.

Kazdin, A. E. and Hartmann, D. P. (1978). The simultaneous-treatment design. *Behavior Therapy, 9*, 912–922.

Kelly, G. A. (1955). *The psychology of personal constructs.* New York: Norton.

Kendall, G., Hrycaiko, D., Martin, G. L. and Kendall, T. (1990). The effects of an imagery rehearsal, relaxation, and self-talk package on basketball game performance. *Journal of Sport & Exercise Psychology, 12*, 157–166.

Kenny, D. A. and Judd, C. M. (1986). Consequences of violating the independence assumption in analysis of variance. *Psychological Bulletin, 99*, 422–431.

Kerr, J. H. (1997). *Motivation and emotion in sport.* Hove, East Sussex: Psychology Press.

Kerr, J. H. (1999). The role of aggression and violence in sport: A rejoinder to the ISSP position stand. *The Sport Psychologist, 13*, 83–88.

Kerr, J. H. (2002). Issues in aggression and violence in sport: The ISSP position stand revisited. *The Sport Psychologist, 16*, 68–78.

Kerr, J. H. (2005). *Rethinking aggression and violence in sport.* Abingdon: Routledge.

Kinugasa, T., Cerin, E. and Hooper, S. (2004). Single-subject research designs and data analyses for assessing elite athletes' conditioning. *Sports Medicine, 34*, 1035–1050.

Kirschenbaum, D. S., Owens, D. D. and O'Connor, E. A. (1998). Smart golf: Preliminary evaluation of a simple, yet comprehensive, approach to improving and scoring the mental game. *The Sport Psychologist, 12*, 271–282.

Komaki, J. and Barnett, F. T. (1977). A behavioral approach to coaching football: Improving the play execution of the offensive backfield on a youth football team. *Journal of Applied Behavior Analysis, 10*, 657–664.

Koop, S. and Martin, G.L. (1983). A coaching strategy to reduce swimming stroke errors with beginning age group swimmers. *Journal of Applied Behavior Analysis, 16*, 447–460.

Kottler, J. A. (2001). *Making changes.* Philadelphia: Brunner-Routledge.

Krane, V., Greenleaf, C. A. and Snow, J. (1997). Reaching for gold and the price of glory: A motivational case study of an elite gymnast. *The Sport Psychologist, 11*, 53–71.

Kratochwill, T. R. (2007). Preparing psychologists for evidence-based school practice: Lessons learned and challenges ahead. *American Psychologist, 62*, 843–845.

Kratochwill, T. R. and Levin, J. R. (2010). Enhancing the scientific credibility of single-case intervention research: Randomization to the rescue. *Psychological Methods, 15*, 124–144.

Kratochwill, T. R., Mott, S. E. and Dodson, C. L. (1984). Case study and single-case research in clinical and applied psychology. In A. S. Bellack (ed.) *Research methods in clinical psychology* (pp. 55–99). Oxford: Pergamon Press.

Kremer, J. and Moran, A. (2008). Swifter, higher, stronger: The history of sport psychology. *The Psychologist, 21*, 740–742.

Lambert, S., Moore, D. W. and Dixon, R. S. (1999). Effects of locus of control on performance under individual-set and coach-determined goal conditions in gymnastics. *Journal of Applied Sport Psychology, 11*, 72–82.

Latham, G. and Locke, E. A. (2002). Building a practically useful theory of goal setting and task motivation. *American Psychologist, 57*, 705–717.

Lavallee, D., Williams, J. and Jones, M. V. J. (2008). Cognitive strategies. In D. Lavallee, J. Williams and M. V. J. Jones (eds) *Key studies in sport and exercise psychology* (pp. 191–203). New York: McGraw-Hill.

Leitenberg, H. (1973). The use of single-case methodology in psychotherapy research. *Journal of Abnormal Psychology, 82*, 87–101.

Lerner, B., Ostrow, A., Yura, M. and Etzel, E. (1996). The effects of goal setting and imagery training programs on the free throw performance of female basketball players. *The Sport Psychologist, 10*, 382–397.

Leslie, J. and O'Reilly, M. F. (1999). *Behavior analysis: Foundations and applications to psychology.* Amsterdam: Harwood.

Lindsay, P., Maynard, I. and Thomas, O. (2005). Effects of hypnosis on flow states and cycling performance. *The Sport Psychologist, 19*, 164–177.

Linton, M. (1975). Memory for real-world events. In D. A. Norman and D. E. Rumelhart (eds), *Explorations in cognition* (pp. 376–404). San Francisco: Freeman.

Luiselli, J. K. (2000). Cueing, demand fading, and positive reinforcement to establish self-feeding and oral consumption in a child with chronic food refusal. *Behavior Modification, 24*, 348–358.

McCarthy, P. J., Jones, M. V., Harwood, C. G. and Davenport, L. (2010). Using goal-setting to enhance positive affect among junior multievent athletes. *Journal of Clinical Sport Psychology, 4*, 53–68.

McDougall, D. (1998). Research on self-management techniques used by students with disabilities in general education settings: A descriptive review. *Remedial and Special Education, 19*, 310–320.

McDougall, D. (2005). The range-bound changing-criterion design. *Behavioral Interventions, 20*, 129–137.

McDougall, D. (2006). The distributed criterion design. *Journal of Behavioral Education, 15*, 236–246.

McDougall, D. and Smith, D. (2006). Recent innovations in small-N designs for research and practice in professional school counseling. *Professional School Counseling, 9*, 392–400.

McDougall, D., Smith, G., Black, R. and Rumrill, P. (2005). Recent innovations in small-N designs for rehabilitation research: An extension of Cowan, Hennessey, Vierstra, and Rumrill. *Journal of Vocational Rehabilitation, 10*, 197–205.

McDougall, D., Hawkins, J., Brady, M. and Jenkins, A. (2006). Recent innovations in the changing criterion design: Implications for research and practice in special education. *Journal of Special Education, 40*, 2–15.

McDougall, D., Skouge, J., Farrell, C. A. and Hoff, K. (2006). Research on self-management techniques used by students with disabilities in general education settings: A promise fulfilled? *Journal of the American Academy of Special Education Professionals*, Summer, *40*, 36–73.

Mace, R. D. (1990). Cognitive behavioral interventions in sport. In G. Jones and L. Hardy (eds) *Stress and performance in sport* (pp. 203–230). Chichester: Wiley.

Mace, R. D. and Carroll, D. (1985). The control of anxiety in sport: Stress inoculation training prior to abseiling. *International Journal of Sport Psychology, 16*, 165–175.

Mace, F. C. and Kratochwill, T. R. (1986). The individual subject in behavior analysis research. In J. Valsiner (eds) *The individual subject and scientific psychology: Perspectives on individual differences* (pp. 153–180). New York: Plenum Press.

Mace, R., Eastman, C. and Carroll, D. (1987). The effects of stress inoculation training on gymnastics performance on the pommelled horse: A case study. *Behavioral Psychotherapy, 15*, 272–279.

McGonigle, J. J., Rojahn, J., Dixon, J. and Strain, P. S. (1987). Multiple treatment interference in the alternating treatments design as a function of the intercomponent interval length. *Journal of Applied Behavior Analysis, 20*, 171–178.

McKenzie, T. L. and Rushall, B. S. (1974). Effects of self-recording on attendance and performance in a competitive swimming training environment. *Journal of Applied Behavior Analysis, 7*, 199–206.

McKenzie, T. L. and Liskevych, T. N. (1983). Using the multi-element baseline design to examine motivation in volleyball training. In G. L. Martin and D. Hrycaiko (eds) Behavior modification and coaching: Principles, procedures, and research (pp. 203–212). Springfield, IL: Charles C Thomas.

Macmillan, M. (2000). Restoring Phineas Gage: A 150th retrospective. *Journal of the History of the Neurosciences, 9*, 46–66.

McNemar, Q. (1940). Sampling in psychological research. *Psychological Bulletin, 37*, 331–365.

Marlow, C., Bull, S., Heath, B. and Shambrook, C. J. (1998). The use of a single case design to investigate the effect of a pre-performance routine on the water polo penalty shot. *Journal of Science and Medicine in Sport, 1*, 143–155.

Martens, R. (1987). Science, knowledge, and sport psychology. *The Sport Psychologist, 1*, 29–55.

Martens, R., Burton, D., Vealey, R. S., Bump, L. A. and Smith, D. E. (1990). Development and validation of the Competitive State Anxiety Inventory – 2. In R. Martens, R. S. Vealey and D. Burton (eds) *Competitive anxiety in sport* (pp. 117–190). Champaign, IL: Human Kinetics.

Martin, G. and Hrycaiko, D. (1983). Effective behavioral coaching: What's it all about? *Journal of Sport Psychology, 5*, 8–20.

Martin, G. L. and Pear, J. J. (2003). *Behavior modification: What it is and how to do it* (7th edn). Upper Saddle River, NJ: Prentice Hall.

Martin, G. L., Thompson, K. and Regehr, K. (2004). Studies using single-subject designs in sport psychology: 30 years of research. *The Behavior Analyst, 27*, 263–280.

Martin, G. L., Vause, T. and Schwartzman, L. (2005). Experimental studies of psychological interventions with athletes in competitions: Why so few? *Behavior Modification, 29*, 616–641.

Maslow, A. H. (1966). *The psychology of science.* Chicago: Henry Regnery.

Mather, G. (2009). *Foundations of sensation and perception* (2nd edn). Hove, East Sussex: Psychology Press.

Matyas, T. A. and Greenwood, K. M. (1991). Problems in the estimation of autocorrelation in brief time series and some implications for behavioral data. *Behavioral Assessment, 13*, 137–157.

Mellalieu, S. D., Hanton, S. and Thomas, O. (2009). The effects of a motivational general-arousal imagery intervention upon preperformance symptoms in male rugby union players. *Psychology of Sport and Exercise, 10*, 175–185.

Messagno, C., Marchant, D. and Morris, T. (2008). A pre-performance routine to alleviate choking in 'choking-susceptible' athletes. *The Sport Psychologist, 22*, 439–457.

Miller, D. R. (1960). Motivation and affect. In P. H. Mussen (ed.) *Handbook of research methods in child development* (pp. 688–769). New York: Wiley.

Miltenberger, R. G., Fuqua, R. W. and McKinley, T. (1985). Habit reversal with muscle tics: Replication and component analysis. *Behavior Therapy, 16*, 39–50.

Mook, D. G. (1983). In defence of external invalidity. *American Psychologist, 38*, 379–387.

Mook, D. G. (2001). *Psychological research: The ideas behind the methods.* London: W. W. Norton.

Moran, A. P. (2011). *Sport and exercise psychology: A critical introduction* (2nd edn). Oxford: Routledge.

Morgan, D. L. and Morgan, R. K. (2001). Single-participant research design: Bringing science to managed care. *American Psychologist, 56*, 119–127.

Morgan D. L. and Morgan, R. K. (2009). *Single-case research methods for the behavioral and health science.* London: Sage Publications.

Murphy, G. (1949). *Historical introduction to modern psychology.* New York: Harcourt, Brace.

Nicholls, J. G. (1984). Achievement motivation: Conceptions of ability, subjective experience, task choice, and performance. *Psychological Review, 91*, 328–346.

Nicholls, J. G. (1989). *The competitive ethos and democratic education.* Cambridge, MA: Harvard University Press.

Nunnally, J. C. and Bernstein, I. A. (1994). *Psychometric methods* (3rd edn). New York: McGraw-Hill.

O'Brien, F., Azrin, N. H. and Henson, K. (1969). Increased communication of chronic mental patients by reinforcement and by response priming. *Journal of Applied Behavior Analysis, 2*, 23–29.

Odom, S. L., Brown, W. H., Frey, T., Karasu, N., Smith-Canter, L. L. and Strain, P. S. (2003). Evidence-based practices for young children with autism: Contributions for single-subject design research. *Focus on Autism and Other Developmental Disabilities, 18*, 166–175.

Ollendick, T. H., Shapiro, E. and Barrett, R. P. (1981). Reducing stereotypic behaviors: An analysis of treatment procedures utilizing an alternating treatments design. *Behavior Therapy, 12*, 570–577.

Orme, J. G. (1991). Statistical conclusion validity and single-system designs. *Social Service Review, 65*, 468–491.

Orne, M. T. (1962). On the social psychology of the psychological experiment: With particular reference to demand characteristics and their implications. *American Psychologist, 17*, 776–783

Ottenbacher, K. J. (1986). *Evaluating clinical change: Strategies for occupational and physical therapists*. Baltimore: Williams and Wilkins.

Ottenbacher, K. J. (1990). Clinically relevant designs for rehabilitation research: The idiographic model. *American Journal of Physical Medicine & Rehabilitation, 69*, 286–292.

Ottenbacher, K. J. and Cusick, A. (1991). An empirical investigation of inter-rater agreement for single-subject data using graphs with and without trendlines. *Journal of the Association for Persons with Severe Handicaps, 16*, 48–55.

Parker, R. I. and Brossart, D. F. (2003). Evaluating single-case research data: A comparison of seven statistical methods. *Behavior Therapy, 34*, 189–211.

Parker, R. I. and Hagan-Burke, S. (2007). Useful effect size interpretations for single case research. *Behavior Therapy, 38*, 95–105.

Parker, R. I. and Vannest, K. (2009). An improved effect size for single-case research: Nonoverlap of all pairs. *Behavior Therapy, 40*, 357–367.

Parker, R. I., Cryer, J. and Byrns, G. (2006). Controlling baseline trend in single-case research. *School Psychology Review, 34*, 116–132.

Parker, R. I., Hagan-Burke, S. and Vannest, K. (2007). Percentage of all non-overlapping data (PAND): An alternative to PND. *Journal of Special Education, 40*, 194–204.

Parkin, A. (1999). *Memory: Phenomena, experiment and theory*. Hove, East Sussex: Psychology Press.

Parsonson, B. S. and Baer, D. M. (1978). The analysis and presentation of graphic data. In T. R. Kratochwill (ed.) *Single subject research: Strategies for evaluating change* (pp. 101–165). New York: Academic Press.

Parsonson, B. S. and Baer, D. M. (1986). The graphic analysis of data. In A. Poling and R. W. Fuqua (eds) *Research methods in applied behavior analysis: Issues and advances* (pp. 157–186). New York: Plenum Press.

Parsonson, B. D. and Baer, D. M. (1992). The visual analysis of data, and current research into the stimuli controlling it. In T. R. Kratochwill anad J. R. Levin (eds) *Single-case research designs and analysis: New directions for psychology and education* (pp. 15–41). Hillsdale, NJ: Erlbaum.

Pates, J. K., Maynard, I. and Westbury, A. (2001). The effects of hypnosis on basketball performance. *Journal of Applied Sport Psychology, 13*, 84–102.

Pates, J. K., Oliver, R. and Maynard, I. (2001). The effects of hypnosis on flow states and golf putting performance. *Journal of Applied Sport Psychology, 13*, 341–354.

Perepletchikova, F. and Kazdin, A. E. (2005). Treatment integrity and therapeutic change: Issues and research recommendations. *Clinical Psychology: Science and Practice, 12*, 365–383.

Piaget, J. (1952). *The origins of intelligence in children*. New York: International University Press.

Powell, J. and Hake, D. F. (1971). Positive vs. negative reinforcement: A direct comparison of effects on complex human response. *Psychological Record, 21*, 191–205.

Prapavessis, H., Grove, J. R., McNair, P. J. and Cable, N. T. (1992). Self-regulation training, state anxiety, and sport performance: A psycho-physiological case study. *The Sport Psychologist, 6*, 213–229.

Prentice, D. A. and Miller, D. T. (1992). When small effects are impressive. *Psychological Bulletin, 112*, 160–164.

Primavera, L. H., Allison, D. B. and Alfonso, V. C. (1996). Measurement of dependent variables. In R. D. Franklin, D. B. Allison and B. S. Gorman (eds) *Design and analysis of single-case research* (pp. 41–92). New York: Psychology Press.

Ray, D. C. and Schottelkorb, A. A. (2010). Single-case design: A primer for play therapists. *International Journal of Play Therapy, 19*, 39–53.

Revusky, S. H. (1967). Some statistical treatments compatible with individual organism methodology. *Journal of the Experimental Analysis of Behavior, 10*, 319–330.

Rhymer, K. N., Dittmer, K. L., Skinner, C. H. and Jackson, B. (2000). Combining explicit timing, peer-delivered immediate feedback, positive-practice overcorrection and performance feedback to increase multiplication fluency. *School Psychology Quarterly, 15*, 40–51.

Rosales-Ruiz, J. and Baer, D. M. (1997). Behavioral cusps: A developmental and pragmatic concept for behaviour analysis. *Journal of Applied Behavior Analysis, 30*, 533–544.

Rosenberg, M. L. (1969). The conditions and consequences of evaluation apprehension. In R. Rosenthal and R. S. Rosnow (eds) *Artifact in behavioral research* (pp. 279–349). New York: Academic Press.

Rosenthal, R. and Rosnow, R. L. (1991). *Essentials of behavioral research: Methods and data analysis* (2nd edn). New York: McGraw-Hill.

Rosenthal, R. and Rosnow, R. (2007). *Essentials of behavioral research: Methods and data analysis* (3rd edn). New York: McGraw-Hill.

Rowbury, T. G., Baer, A. M. and Baer, D. M. (1976). Interactions between teacher guidance and contigient access to play in developing preacademic skills of deviant preschool children. *Journal of Applied Behavior Analysis, 9*, 85–104.

Rush, D. B. and Ayllon, T. (1984). Peer behavioral coaching: Soccer. *Journal of Sport Psychology, 6*, 325–334.

Rushall, B. S. and Siedentop, D. (1972). *The development and control of behavior in sport and physical education*. Philadelphia: Lea & Febiger.

Rushall, B. S. and Smith, K. S. (1979). The modification of the quality and quantity of behavior categories in a swimming coach. *Journal of Sport Psychology, 1*, 138–150.

Sacks, O. (1985). *The man who mistook his wife for a hat*. New York: Summit Books.

Sariscsany, M. J., Darst, P. W. and van der Mars, H. (1995). The effects of three teacher supervision patterns on student on-task and skill performance in secondary physical education. *Journal of Teaching in Physical Education, 14*, 179–197.

Schloss, P. J., Sedlak, R. A., Elliot, C. and Smothers, M. (1982). Application of the changing-criterion design in special education. *Journal of Special Education, 16*, 359–367.

Schwartz, R. M. and Garamoni, G. L. (1986). Cognitive assessment: A multibehavior-multimethod-multiperspective approach. *Journal of Psychopathology and Behavioral Assessment, 8*, 185–197.

Schwartz, S. (1987). *Pavlov's heirs: Classic psychology experiments that changed the way we view ourselves*. London: Harper Collins.

Scruggs, T. E. and Mastropieri, M. A. (2001). How to summarize single-participant research: Ideas and applications. *Exceptionality, 9*, 227–244.

Scruggs, T. E., Mastropieri, M. A., Cook, S. and Escobar, C. (1986). Early intervention for children with conduct disorders: A quantitative synthesis of single-subject research. *Behavioral Disorders, 11*, 260–271.

Sears, D. O. (1986). College sophomores in the laboratory: Influences of a narrow data base on social psychology's view of human nature. *Journal of Personality and Social Psychology, 51*, 515–530.

Seligman, M. E. P. (1995). The effectiveness of psychotherapy: The *Consumer Reports* study. *American Psychologist, 50*, 965–974.

Shapiro, E., Kazdin, A. and McGonigle, J. (1982). Multiple treatment interference in the simultaneous or alternating treatments design. *Behavioral Assessment, 4*, 105–115.

Shaughnessy, J. J., Zechmeister, E. B. and Zechmeister, E. B. (2000). *Research methods in psychology* (5th edn). Boston: McGraw-Hill.

Shearer, D., Mellalieu, S., Shearer, C. and Roderique-Davies, G. (2009). The effects of a video-aided imagery intervention upon collective efficacy in an international paralympic wheelchair basketball team. *Journal of Imagery Research in Sport and Physical Activity, 4*, 190–210.

Sidman, M. (1960). *Tactics of scientific research: Evaluating experimental data in psychology*. New York: Basic Books.

Sierra, V., Quera, V. and Solanas, A. (2000). Autocorrelation effect on type 1 error rate of Rvusky's R_n tests: A Monte Carlo study. *Psicologica, 21*, 91–114.

Skinner, B. F. (1966). Operant behavior. In W. K. Honig (ed.) *Operant behavior: Areas of research and application* (pp. 12–32). New York: Apleton-Century-Crofts.

Skinner, C. H. (2004). Single-subject designs: Procedures that allow school psychologists to contribute to the intervention, evaluation, and validation process. *Journal of Applied School Psychology, 20*, 1–10.

Skinner, C. H., Skinner, A. L. and Armstrong, K. J. (2000). Analysis of a client–staff developed shaping program designed to enhance reading persistence in an adult in an adult diagnosed with schizophrenia. *Psychiatric Rehabilitation Journal, 24*, 52–57.

Smith, R. E. (1988). The logic and design of case study research. *The Sport Psychologist, 2*, 1–12.

Smith, R. E. (1989). Applied sport psychology in an age of accountability. *Journal of Applied Sport Psychology, 1*, 166–180.

Smith, R. E. and Smoll, F. L. (1996). Psychological interventions in youth sports. In J. Van Raalte and B. W. Brewer (eds) *Exploring sport and exercise psychology* (pp. 125–141). Washington, DC: American Psychological Association.

Smith, R. E., Smoll, F. L. and Hunt, E. (1977). A system for the behavioral assessment of athletic coaches. *Research Quarterly, 48*, 401–407.

Smith, R. E., Smoll, F. L. and Curtis, B. (1979). Coach effectiveness training: A cognitive behavioral approach to enhancing relationship skills in youth sport coaches. *Journal of Sport Psychology, 1*, 59–75.

Smith, R. E., Smoll, F. L. and Barnett, N. P. (1995). Reduction of children's sport performance anxiety through social support and stress-reduction training for coaches. *Journal of Applied Developmental Psychology, 16*, 125–142.

Smith, R. E., Smoll, F. L. and Christensen, D. S. (1996). Behavioral assessment and interventions in youth sports. *Behavior Modification, 20*, 3–44.

Smith, S. L. and Ward, P. (2006). Behavioral interventions to improve performance in collegiate football. *Journal of Applied Behavior Analysis, 39*, 385–391.

Sprague, J. R. and Horner, R. H. (1992). Covariation within functional response classes: Implications for treatment of severe problem behavior. *Journal of Applied Behavior Analysis, 25*, 735–745.

Stake, R. E. (1988). Case study methods in educational research: Seeking sweet water. In R. M. Jaeger (ed.) *Complementary methods for research in education* (pp. 253–278). Washington, DC: American Educational Research Association.

Stake, R. E. (2000). Case studies. In N. K. Denzin and Y. S. Lincoln (eds) *Handbook of qualitative research* (pp. 435–454). London: Sage.

Strømgren, B. and Kolby, L. J. (1996). The alternating-treatments design: Little used and often confused? *Scandinavian Journal of Behavior Therapy, 25*, 127–138.

Swain, A. and Jones, G. (1995). Effects of goal-setting interventions on selected basketball skills: A single-subject design. *Research Quarterly for Exercise and Sport, 66*, 51–63.

Tankersley, M., Cook, B. G. and Cook, L. (2008). A preliminary examination to identify the presence of quality indicators in single-subject research. *Education and Treatment of Children, 31*, 523–548.

Tenenbaum, G., Stewart, E., Singer, R. N. and Duda, J. (1997). Aggression and violence in sport: An ISSP position stand. *The Sport Psychologist, 11*, 1–7.

Tenenbaum, G., Sacks, D. N., Miller, J. W., Golden, A. S. and Doolin, N. (2000). Aggression and violence in sport: A reply to Kerr's rejoinder. *The Sport Psychologist, 14*, 315–332.

Thelwell, R. C. and Greenlees, I. A. (2001). The effects of a mental skills training package on gymnasium triathlon performance. *The Sport Psychologist, 15*, 127–141.

Thelwell, R. C. and Greenlees, I. A. (2003). Developing competitive endurance performance using mental skills training. *The Sport Psychologist, 17*, 318–337.

Thelwell, R. C., Greenlees, I. and Weston, N. J. V. (2006). Using psychological skills training to develop soccer performance. *Journal of Applied Sport Psychology, 18*, 254–270.

Thomas, J. R. (1980). Half a cheer for Rainer and Daryl. *Journal of Sport Psychology, 2*, 266–267.

Thomas, J. R., Nelson, J. K. and Silverman, S. J. (2005). *Research methods in physical activity* (5th edn). Champaign, IL: Human Kinetics.

Tkachuk, G., Leslie-Toogood, A. and Martin, G. L. (2003). Behavioral assessment in sport psychology. *The Sport Psychologist, 17*, 104–117.

Tolman, C. (ed.) (1991). *Positivism in psychology: Historical and contemporary approaches*. New York: Springer.

Triplett, N. (1898). The dynamogenic factors in pacemaking and competition. *American Journal of Psychology, 9*, 507–533.

Ulman, J. D. and Sulzer-Azaroff, B. (1975). Multielement baseline design in educational research. In E. Ramp and G. Semb (eds) *Behavior analysis: Areas of research and application* (pp. 377–391). Englewood Cliffs, NJ: Prentice-Hall.

Uphill, M. A. and Jones, M. V. (2005). Coping with and reducing the number of careless shots: A case study with a county golfer. *Sport and Exercise Psychology Review, 2*, 14–22.

Vaughan, G. M. and Guerin, B. (1997). A neglected innovator in sports psychology. Norman Triplett and the early history of competitive performance. *International Journal of the History of Sport, 14*, 82–99.

Vealey, R. S. and Walter, S. M. (1994). On target with mental skills: An interview with Darrell Pace. *The Sport Psychologist, 8*, 427–441.

Wacker, D., McMahon, C., Steege, M., Berg, W., Sasso, G. and Melloy, K. (1990). Applications of a sequential alternating treatments design. *Journal of Applied Behavior Analysis, 23*, 333–339.

Walker, H. M. (1929). *Studies in the history of statistical method, with special reference to certain educational problems*. Baltimore: Williams & Wilkins.

Ward, J. (2010). *The student's guide to cognitive neuroscience* (2nd edn). Hove, East Sussex: Psychology Press.

Watson, D., Clarke, L. A. and Tellegen, A. (1988). Development and validation of brief measures of positive and negative affect: The PANAS scales. *Journal of Personality and Social Psychology, 54*, 1063–1070.

Watson, J. B. and Rayner, R. (1920). Conditioned emotional reactions. *Journal of Experimental Psychology, 3*, 1–14.

Weis, L. and Hall, R. V. (1971). Modifcation of cigarette smoking through avoidance of punishment. In R. V. Hall (ed.) *Managing behavior: Behavior modification applications in school and home* (pp. 77–103). Lawrence, KS: H & H Enterprises.

Weston, N. (2008). Performance profiling. In A. M. Lane (ed.) *Sport and exercise psychology: Topics in applied psychology* (pp. 91–107). London: Hodder Education.

White, O. R. (1971). *A glossary of behavioral terminology*. Champaign, IL: Research Press.

White, O. R. (1974). *The 'split-middle': A 'quickie' method of trend estimation*. Seattle, WA: University of Washington, Experimental Educational Unit, Child Development and Mental Retardation Center.

White, O. R. (1987). Some comments concerning 'the quantitative synthesis of single-subject research'. *Remedial and Special Education, 8,* 34–39.

White, O. R. (2005). Trend lines. In G. Sugai and R. Horner (eds) *Encyclopedia of behavior modification and cognitive behavior therapy* (Vol. 3) (pp. 1589–1593). London: Sage Publications.

Whitehead, T. N. (1938). *The industrial worker: A statistical study of human relations in a group of manual workers*. Cambridge, MA: Harvard University Press.

Wolery, M. and Harris, S. R. (1982). Interpreting results of single-subject research designs. *Physical Therapy, 62,* 445–452.

Wolery, M., Bailey, D. B. and Sugai, G. M. (1988). *Effective teaching: Principles and procedures of applied behavior analysis with exceptional students*. Boston: Allyn & Bacon.

Wolf, M. M. (1978). Social validity: The case for subjective measurement or how applied behavior analysis is finding its heart. *Journal of Applied Behavior Analysis, 11,* 203–214.

Wolko, K. L., Hrycaiko, D. W. and Martin, G. L. (1993). A comparison of two self-management packages to standard coaching for improving practice performance of gymnasts. *Behavior Modification, 17,* 209–223.

Wollman, N. (1986). Research on imagery and motor performance: Three methodological suggestions. *Journal of Sport Psychology, 8,* 135–138.

Woods, D. W., Miltenberger, R. G. and Lumley, V. A. (1996). Sequential application of major habit reversal components to treat motor tics in children. *Journal of Applied Behavior Analysis, 29,* 483–493.

Yukelson, D. P. (2010). Communicating effectively. In J. M. Williams (ed.) *Applied sport psychology: Personal growth to peak performance* (6th ed) (pp. 149–168). New York: McGraw-Hill.

Zaichkowsky, L. D. (1980). Single-case experimental designs and sport psychology research. In C. H. Nadeau, W. R. Halliwell, K. M. Newell and G. C. Roberts (eds) *Psychology of motor behavior and sport* (pp. 171–179). Champaign, IL: Human Kinetics.

Zaichkowsky, L. and Takenaka, K. (1993). Optimizing arousal level. In R. N. Singer, M. Murphey and L. K. Tennant (eds), *Handbook of research on sport psychology* (pp. 511–527). New York: Macmillan.

Zhan, S. and Ottenbacher, K. J. (2001). Single-subject experimental designs for disability research. *Disability and Rehabilitation, 23,* 1–8.

INDEX